How to Sit
Your Body at Work

Also available from Balance Arts Center:

Working with Less Stress and More Energy
An audio guide to use in your workplace for more ease and focus on the job

How to Sit Poster
Remind yourself how to maintain your best sitting balance every time you look up from your computer or go to the water cooler with this ergonomics poster.

To order visit www.balanceartcenter.com

How to Sit
Your Body at Work

A guide to sitting at your workstation
based on the Alexander Technique

Ann Rodiger
Founder of the Balance Arts Center

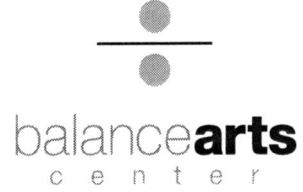

www.balanceartscenter.com

Acknowledgments

Thank you to F. M. Alexander for the guiding principles of psychophysical education that are the fundamental organizing aspects of all we do. And thank you to all of my students who have provided a practical laboratory through which to learn how to apply these principles. Everyone has a unique situation and story. Each student illuminates a new facet of the human element in the ergonomics picture.

Cover Design, Graphics, and Layout: Michael Stewart
Editorial Consultants: Karen Braga, Rebecca Brooks, Emily Halpern, Kathleen Moore, Sarah White-Ayon
Photo Subjects: Tom Baird, Sarah White-Ayon
Photography: Donna Fields

© 2011 Balance Arts Center, LLC

All rights reserved. No part of this publication may be reproduced, stored in a retrieval system, or transmitted, in any form or by any means, electronic, photocopying, recording, or otherwise, without the prior written permission of the publisher.

Ann Rodiger
Balance Arts Center, LLC © 2010
New York City, NY USA
www.balanceartscenter.com

Published by
Dog Ear Publishing
4010 W. 86th Street, Ste H
Indianapolis, IN 46268
www.dogearpublishing.net

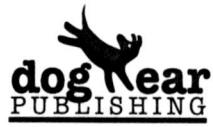

ISBN: 978-160844-788-6

This book is printed on acid-free paper.

Please consult with a physician if you have an injury. This book is not intended to substitute for medical consultation, advice or treatment. The author and publisher disclaim any and all liability arising directly or indirectly from the use of any information contained in this book.

"Change involves carrying out an activity against the habit of life."
—F. M. Alexander

contents

Introduction		**1-2**
Chapter 1:	The Basics – Overview of Elements	**3-5**
	WHO: You – The Human Factor	3
	WHAT: The Physical Setup	3
	WHERE: At Your Desk or Workstation	4
	HOW: Attention – Change Your Habits	4
	WHEN: Often	5
	WHY: Feel Better and Be More Productive	5
Chapter 2:	Harmful Postures	**6-11**
Chapter 3:	The Physical Setup	**12-16**
	Desk	14
	Chair	14
	Screen	15
	Keyboard / Mouse	16
	Environmental Suggestions	16
Chapter 4:	How to Change Your Patterns	**17-23**
	Step 1: Observe / Identify Stimuli	19
	Step 2: Alert Pause / Active Non-doing	21
	Step 3: Balance and Redirect Yourself / Make a Choice	22
	Step 4: Move with Ease / Respond	23
Chapter 5:	Sample Activity – Answering the Phone	**24-26**
Chapter 6:	Step 3 Expanded: What to Think and Notice	**27-43**
	Starting at the Top: Head and Neck	27
	How You See: Eyes	30
	Jaw and Tongue	31
	Your Head Leads Your Torso: Length and Width Of Your Back	33
	Ongoing Motion: Breathing	34
	Connect to the Chair: Pelvis	35
	Connect to the Floor: Legs and Feet	37
	Typing: Arms, Wrists, and Hands	38
	Words on the Screen: Pressure / Force on the Keyboard	41
	Mousing Around: Hands and Mouse	42

Chapter 7:	Working at a Laptop Computer	**44-45**
Chapter 8:	Working on the Bed	**46**
Chapter 9:	Writing with Pen and Paper	**47-48**
Chapter 10:	What to Think When...	**49-50**
	Your Back Aches	49
	Your Neck Hurts	49
	Your Shoulders Ache	49
	Your Eyes Are Tired	50
	Your Wrists and Hands Are Sore	50
	Your Feet Hurt	50
	You Can't Think Anymore	50
Chapter 11:	Recuperation on the Job	**51-52**
	Warning Signs that You Need a Break	51
	Short Breaks	51
	Longer Breaks	52
Chapter 12:	Getting to Work	**53-54**
	Sitting in the Car	53
	Sitting on the Bus, Train, or Subway	53
	Walking to Work	54
Chapter 13:	The Alexander Technique	**55-56**
Chapter 14:	Review / Ideas to Remember	**57**
Chapter 15:	Concepts of the Alexander Technique	**58-59**
Chapter 16:	Supplementary Information	**60-63**
	F. M. Alexander	60
	The Balance Arts Center	60
	Recommended Readings and Resources	61

introduction

This book addresses the human element of office ergonomics – how you interact with your workspace environment. You will learn how to work at your desk in a way that allows your body to support and enhance your thinking, focus, speed on the keyboard, and overall productivity at work.

Your goal, with the help of this book, is to build a mental and physical awareness that allows you to reduce and eliminate stress, excess tensions, and thoughts that keep you from being at your best. You can keep tensions from accumulating during the day by understanding how to maintain a sense of balance and ease throughout your entire being.

This will reduce your risk of injury and increase your safety on the job. Many ideas will be presented here about how you interface with the variables in your sitting work environment. Explore these ideas and see where they take you.

You will not limit or change your work activities. You will simply change the way you perceive and perform them. Your conscious awareness and self-knowledge are the keys to creating this change in action.

When combined with a good ergonomic setup, the Alexander Technique will provide you with a means of working that will increase the duration of your work sessions and your longevity on the job.

The principles you will learn in this book are based on the Alexander Technique. The Alexander Technique teaches a way to discover, understand, and refine your knowledge of how you move and interact with your environment. You will find that your coordination while walking, exercising, and enjoying leisure activities will improve due to the attention you give to yourself at work.

Through building an awareness of your thinking and core movement patterns and learning how to fundamentally change them for the better, you will experience improvements in your physical and mental health and well-being.

When you work well, you avoid:
- Injury
- Stress
- Excess tension
- Stiff and sore muscles at the end of the day
- Eye strain
- Headaches
- Backaches
- Fatigue
- Breathing problems
- Repetitive Stress Injury (RSI)
- Vocal stress and strain
- Neck and shoulder tension

When you work well, you will enjoy:
- Clearer vision
- Clearer thinking
- Freer breathing
- Ease in your joints
- Clearer and stronger voice
- More energy at work
- Ability to stay calm in stressful situations
- More energy at the end of the day

chapter one
The Basics – Overview of Elements

An overview of the elements who, what, where, how, when, why, is useful so you can immediately see how you are working with your whole being. These basics will be given more attention in the following pages.

You will not learn a set of "exercises" or "postures" that you can do and then forget about for the rest of the day. You will learn a balanced way of working and an awareness that you can use for a long time and in many settings.

WHO: You–The Human Factor

The human element is the factor that is most frequently left out of the ergonomic equation. You are an integral factor in the ergonomic setup and its functioning. You could have the best, most expensive setup available and yet still have aches and pains from working at your workstation. By refining how you move and how you think about moving, you can make a difference in the outcome of your workday.

You will discover that you have more choices in how you work than you might have thought. You will find that your active participation in the process will make an enormous difference in your well-being.

WHAT: The Physical Setup

Having a setup that allows you to work optimally is extremely helpful in maintaining good health and a pain-free body.

Each of us has a unique body with our own proportions, so we need to tailor our equipment setup to fit our own needs. You may spend quite a bit of time working, so making the appropriate adjustments to your setup will substantially increase your level of comfort and productivity. The more options you have to adjust your setup, the better. The variables in a work setup include desk and chair heights as well as placement of monitor, keyboard, mouse, and other objects you use frequently.

Would you ride a bicycle or drive a car that was misaligned so you had to compensate constantly just to keep the bike or car going straight down the road? Not likely. The same thing should be true at your desk. It doesn't make sense to work in a situation that requires you to adjust and adapt constantly in ways that pull you off balance and pull your focus off your work.

WHERE: At Your Desk or Workstation

The ideas presented here are specifically related to the activities you perform at your workstation. You will learn to find ways of sitting that will help with typing, handwriting, answering the phone, working with files, and so on.

The principles presented relate to and apply to all the actions you perform throughout the day. Use your work activities and setup as a laboratory for discovering how to improve all of your activities.

HOW: Attention–Change Your Habits

You are going to learn to pay attention in a way that will change your work habits for the better. This process of learning and building awareness requires focusing on yourself. As you become aware of the various activities and stimuli that are in your sitting environment, you will be able to attend to them in a way that gives you more choice in your response. You will learn to recognize the choices you are making currently that may be detrimental and direct yourself to make new choices. Often the current choices are unconscious and need to be brought forward into your awareness. Sometimes seemingly small unconscious habits have a very large effect on the outcome of your day.

one: the basics

Learning to pay attention to your habitual movements and patterns will not take your attention or time away from your work. You will see very shortly that even a few new ideas can result in changes in how you feel and work.

WHEN: Often

The more you pay attention to the ideas presented in this book the more quickly you will improve and discover the benefits of this new way of working. You will find that noticing what you do and giving yourself directions will become an integral and integrated part of your work routine. At first it might seem to you that you could drive yourself crazy by constantly paying attention to these ideas. If that is the case, incorporate the process slowly into your work routine. Sticking with the process at whatever pace you choose will be well worth it.

WHY: To Feel Better and Be More Productive

The freer and more balanced you are in your body, the better you think and feel. The better you think and feel the more focused you can be. And the more focused and clear you are, the more productive you will be without accumulating new tensions. As you acquire new habits you will enhance your thinking and productivity. You will find yourself on an upward spiral toward ease and lightness.

You are learning a process that helps prevent stress and injury. This is a process of refined balance and can result in new habitual ways of moving and being. It will lead you to thinking that is creative and movement that is coordinated and easy.

chapter two
Harmful Postures

Many of us have a combination of the harmful postures described in this chapter. Use the tips below each illustration of a harmful posture to identify how you can begin to help yourself change.

Following the instructions will clarify your understanding and expand your knowledge. How to change your habits and what to think will be explored in the next chapters.

These initial tips will help you begin to undo your typical working habits and prepare you for the next step —- a more refined awareness of your current habits and a process of working better. You will discover a fuller breath, learn an expanded movement vocabulary, and sense more freedom in the movements themselves.

As you adjust your setup, set YOURSELF up first and THEN adjust your environment to fit YOU rather than adapting yourself to an existing environment.

It is well worth the 15, 20, 30 minutes it will take to adjust your chair, desk height, screen, keyboard, and the other work items in your environment.

two: harmful postures

Harmful Posture No. 1

Fig. 1 Perching up on chair

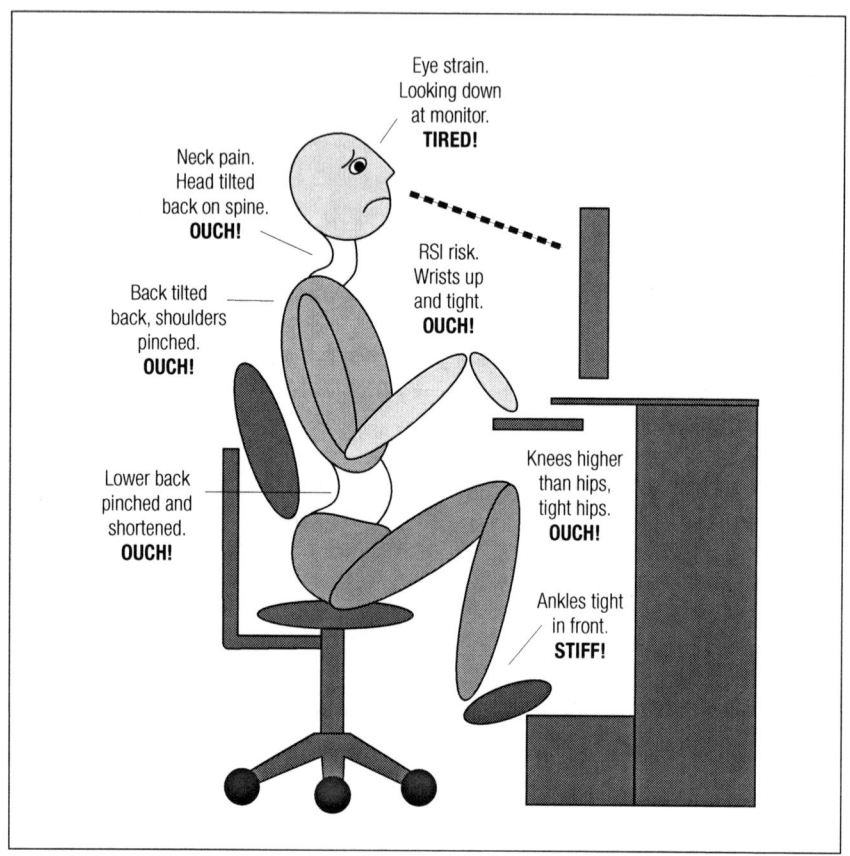

Tips:
- Free your neck.
- Lengthen your neck (without reaching up with your head).
- Balance your head on your spine.
- Let your head lead your whole back, including your spine, up into length and width.
- Continue to sense your body weight on the chair.
- Look straight ahead or slightly down.
- Let your wrists be in front of and horizontal to or below your elbows.
- Let your hands be an extension of your lower arms.
- Put your knees horizontal to or below your hip joints.
- Place your feet flat on the floor.
- BREATHE.

Harmful Posture No. 2
Fig. 2 Curving forward

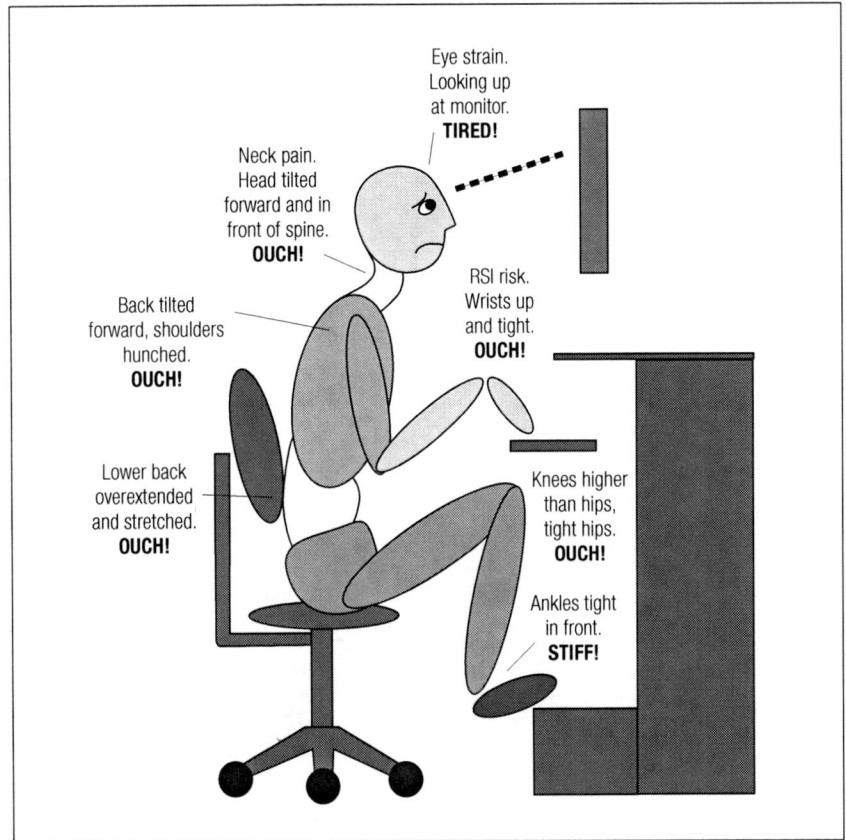

Tips:
- Free your neck.
- Bring your head back above your pelvis.
- Let your head lead your whole back, including your spine, up into length and width.
- Allow for width in the front of your chest and across your shoulder girdle.
- Allow for a lower back curve.
- Sit on your sit bones (the end of your torso).
- Look straight ahead.
- Let your wrists be in front of and horizontal to or below your elbows
- Let your hands be an extension of your lower arms.
- Put your knees horizontal to or below your hip joints.
- Place your feet flat on the floor.
- BREATHE.

two: harmful postures

Harmful Posture No. 3
Fig. 3 Leaning back

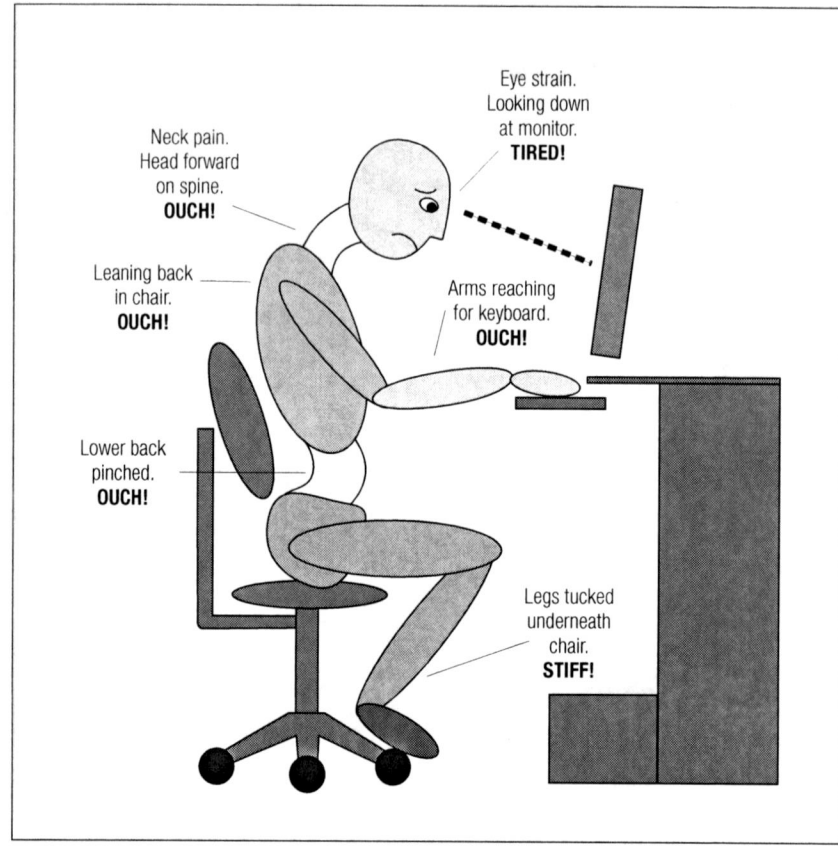

Tips:
- Free your neck.
- Bring your head forward over above your pelvis.
- Allow for curves in both your neck and lower back.
- Let your head lead your whole back, including your spine, up into length and width.
- Sit on your sit bones (the end of your torso).
- Look straight ahead.
- Allow your elbows to bend.
- Allow your elbows to hang below your shoulders.
- Let your wrists be in front of and horizontal to or below your elbows.
- Let your hands be an extension of your lower arms.
- Place your feet flat on the floor.
- BREATHE.

Harmful Posture No. 4
Fig. 4 One-legged perch

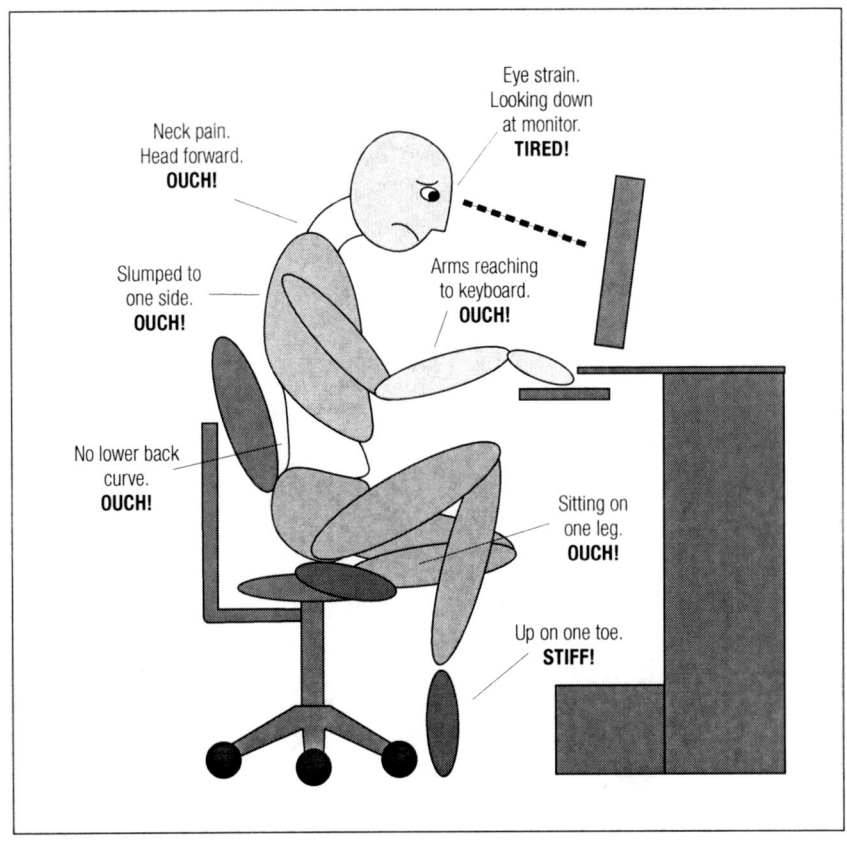

Tips:
- Free your neck.
- Place both feet flat on the floor.
- Sit on both sit bones evenly.
- Let your head lead your whole back up into length and width.
- Let both sides of your torso lengthen evenly.
- BREATHE.

Harmful Posture No. 5

Fig. 5 Lateral imbalance

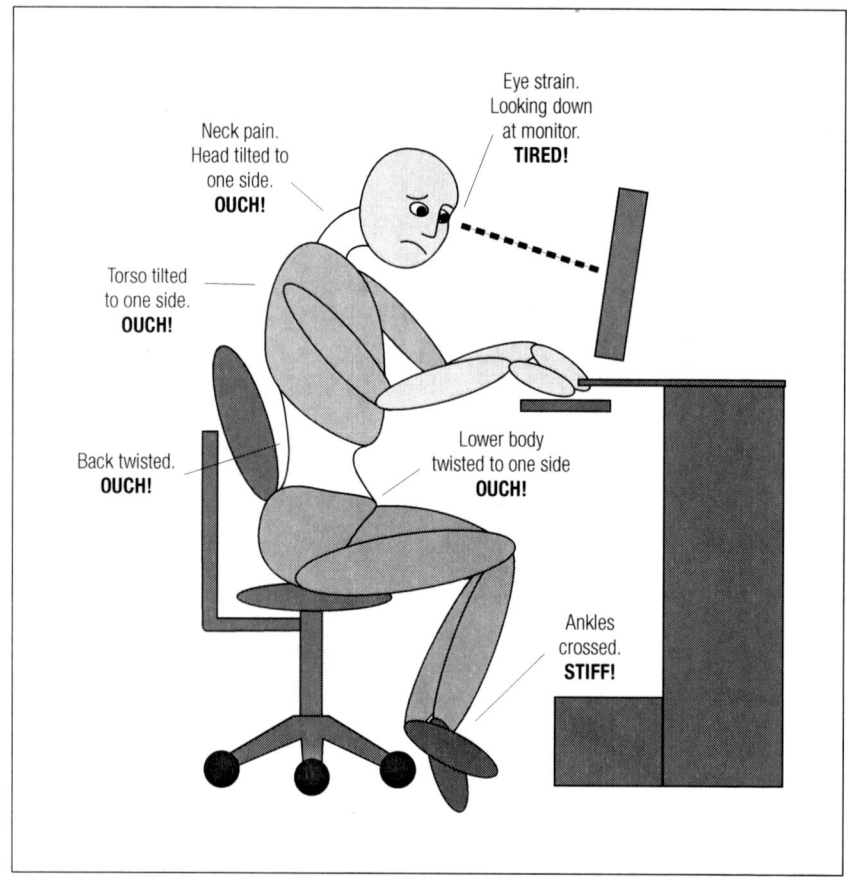

Tips:
- Free your neck.
- Face forward with your whole body (untwist your lower body).
- Uncross your legs.
- Place both feet flat on the floor.
- Sit on both sit bones evenly.
- Let your head lead your whole back up into length and width.
- Let both sides of your torso lengthen evenly.
- BREATHE.

chapter three
The Physical Setup

Now that you have a good start at organizing yourself in your chair, set up your computer, desk, mouse, and footrest (if needed). The setup process itself will help guide you toward and encourage you to experience and maintain your best balance.

Remember that you are looking for a situation that allows you to balance and move, find movement flow within your posture, and motion in stillness.

Your work may require you to do several different functions such as typing, writing by hand, and reading. Make sure you have a proper setup to do each task. You might want to dedicate a different part of your desk to each activity.

Also make sure your setup allows you to turn to the side, stand up and sit down easily.

Approach your setup as if you, rather than the desk or chair, are the constant or "fixed" entity in the equation. Fit the furniture to your individual lengths and preferences. You may be working with what seem to be permanent fixtures in the environment but there are always ways to rearrange what is given to you. The process may seem like a puzzle where you adjust one element and then find that you have to adjust another, and then another.

Take the necessary time to get your setup right for you. This may ultimately require calling maintenance or service personnel to obtain more appropriate furniture or move existing items. It is time well spent as you will be much more productive due to the clear thinking and better focus that accompany moving with ease.

three: the physical setup

An ergonomic setup that suits you might look like this:

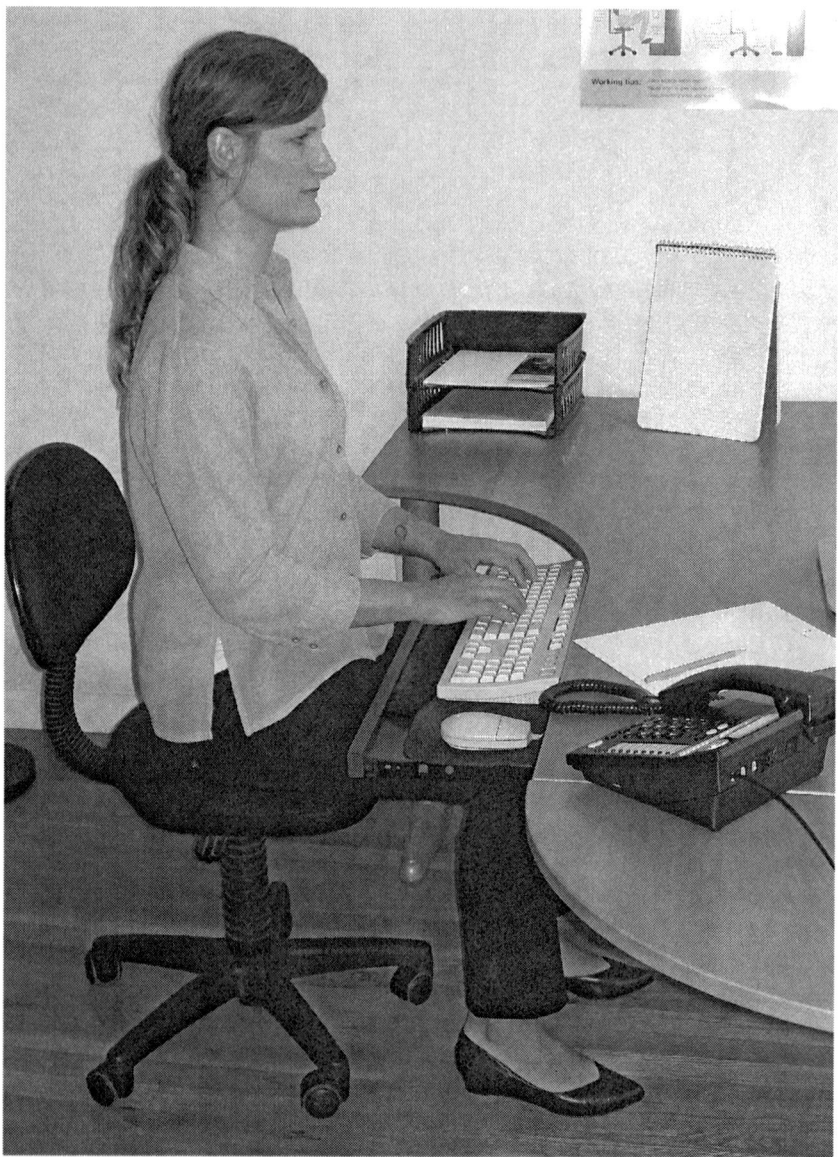

Fig. 6 This setup allows for a balanced posture.

three: the physical setup

Desk

Often the desk is the least variable and hardest to adjust piece of furniture in an office setup, so we will start here. First orient your forearms to your desk surface and keyboard. Your forearms should be horizontal to the desk surface or slanted so your wrists are slightly below the elbows. Build the rest of your setup from there.

Consider these optimal conditions when choosing a desk for yourself:
- Your knees and thighs fit easily underneath the desk. If you use a keyboard tray take that into consideration when deciding on the height of the desk surface.
- You can move your legs side to side and not feel "trapped" by file cabinets or other items.
- There is enough surface area for all the different tasks you will do at the desk, e.g., typing and writing by hand.
- Phones and working materials are within easy reach.

Suggestions:
- Find an orientation for the desk in your office area that feels good to you.
- Orient your chair so you can look mostly forward while interacting with colleagues, e.g. you don't have to twist around constantly to view visitors and colleagues.
- Position filing cabinets so that you can access the contents easily.
- Orient the desk to avoid glare in your eyes.

Chair

Find a chair that fits your body in the following ways:
- The lumbar support in the backrest matches your own lower back curve.
- Your thighs are parallel to the floor.
- Your knees may be slightly below the hip level.
- The backs of your knees are in front of the edge of the seat.
- Your lower legs are directly down from the knees.
- Your feet are flat on the floor or footrest.

Suggestions:
- Spend time finding the right chair for you.
- Choose a chair that encourages you to sit fairly upright.
- Have a firm sitting surface so you can sense your sit bones on the chair.

three: the physical setup

- A firm cushion or wedge may make the hard surface of the chair seat more comfortable.
- Make sure the seat surface does not slant backward.
- Be sure the chair or cushion does not cut off circulation at the back of your thighs.

Armrests:
- Are not necessary.
- If you have armrests make sure they are at a level that allows you to have free movement of your arms and shoulders.

Footrest:
- Avoid dangling feet.
- Use it to keep feet flat on the floor or on a footrest.

Screen

If your main computer is a laptop and you spend many hours a day at the computer, invest in an external monitor and/or external keyboard. This will allow you to find the optimal setup for yourself.

Make sure the screen is:
- Positioned so the top of the screen is at your eye level.
- 18 – 28 inches away from your eyes.
- Close enough to you that you don't have to lean your head forward to read it.

Suggestions:
- Pay particular attention to the screen angle and placement if you wear bifocal or trifocal glasses. Make sure you don't tilt your head backward and pull your chin up to view the screen.
- Get a special pair of glasses for computer work if that helps you see more easily.
- If you find yourself squinting make the font size larger. You can always reduce it when you are finished reading a document.
- Adjust the brightness of the screen to best suit your eyes.

three: the physical setup

Keyboard/Mouse

Find a setup that allows for the following:
- Wide and relaxed shoulders.
- Elbows hanging directly down from your shoulders.
- Wrists and hands horizontal and slightly below the elbows.
- Mouse pad at the same level as the keyboard and within easy reach.

Suggestions:
- Find a keyboard where you can use minimal force when contacting the keys.
- External keyboards can be very useful in creating the best ergonomic setup with a laptop.
- If you have wrist pain, it may be well worth the few hours it takes to become accustomed to an ergonomic keyboard – one that splits the two sides of the keyboard. (Ergonomic keyboards allow the wrists to be longer so the forearm and hand are in a more continuous line.)
- Wrist pads may help you keep your wrists elongated.
- Take a typing class or get a typing program if you are a "hunt-and-peck" keyboard operator.
- Find the right mouse size for you. Choose a mouse that you can hold lightly, that glides across the mouse pad easily, and that allows you to move your wrist and fingers easily.

Environmental Suggestions

The physical setup is critical and so is the rest of your environment.
- Find the best orientation for your setup within the room or work environment. This may be different from that chosen by the previous occupant of the workspace.
- Make sure your computer screen is clean and easy to read.
- Adjust the monitor brightness and contrast to suit you.
- Adjust the light in the room to reduce glare from windows and overhead lights.
- Avoid intense light sources in your field of vision.
- Keep the environment at a comfortable temperature and avoid drafts.
- Find a place free from distracting noises.

chapter four
How to Change Your Patterns

You have started to address your posture, your environment, and the objects in your workspace. It is time to shift your focus on how to interact with your setup. Awareness and self-observation are the key.

The process you are about to learn will help you identify your thinking and the movement habits that cause you stress, strain, and pain, or habits that are potentially injurious. You will discover options and choices to help you leave behind those less than optimal habits.

The process itself is fairly simple. Through it you will build and refine your mental and kinesthetic (bodily felt sense) awareness. You participate by observing, monitoring, and directing your thinking and actions. Think of this as an exploration and refinement of your movement habits at work.

You may already be aware of what you are doing and have no idea what to do about it. You are about to learn how to accomplish a task in a new way.

Clue: The solution to your discomfort may not be to focus directly on that area or spot where you feel sensation. For instance, focusing on where your back hurts may not solve your back pain. A change in the use of your whole body is much more effective.

Another way to describe what you are doing is that you are learning to work with:

STIMULUS – ACTIVE PAUSE - CHOICE – RESPONSE

The STIMULUS is anything internal and/or external that comes your way, such as:
- Striking the keyboard.
- Moving the mouse.
- Sitting down in the chair.

- Creating a sentence on the screen.
- Standing up from the chair.
- Listening to someone speak to you.

The ACTIVE PAUSE is giving yourself a moment before you take action to consciously inhibit and not do what you normally do with the given stimulus. This is the moment before the response in which you decide NOT TO DO your normal response. You ACTIVELY PAUSE to keep yourself from repeating what you have been doing unconsciously.

The CHOICE, which will take place during the active pause, is where your thinking comes into the picture. You choose a process of direction and balance to go with instead of moving automatically. You allow your body to accommodate to the directions you are giving it.

In RESPONSE you allow the activity to take place according to the directions and choices you have made. You are allowing for unfamiliar and new sensations and results.

Building General Awareness

Before you get to the specifics, observe yourself at work and see what you notice. Look at your whole body balance and posture even if you are experiencing discomfort in only one particular area.

Observations:
- Find an overall sense of your body. Do you feel heavy, fatigued, buoyant, light? Something else?
- Does this change throughout the workday?
- Do you notice aches and pains anywhere?
- Notice your breathing pattern. How far down into your body do you sense your breath? (Chest, abdomen, pelvis, feet?)
- When are you the most comfortable?
- What stimuli cause you to freeze or contract?
- Are you aware of your body when you are thinking or speaking to someone?

four: how to change your patterns

At the Computer:
- Where is your head in relation to the screen?
- What part of your pelvis makes contact with the chair seat?
- How much force do you use to type on the keyboard?

When You Are Writing by Hand:
- Where is your head in relation to the paper?
- How much force are you using to hold the pen or pencil?
- How much force are you using to move the pen or pencil across the page?
- Where is your arm in relation to the desk?

The following steps 1-4 will guide you in expanding and deepening your awareness. They will help you work with specific stimuli and they can be applied to any task you do.

Step 1: Observe / Identify Stimuli

Notice how you want to start a specific activity such as getting up from your desk, reaching for the phone or bringing your hands to the keyboard. Find the moment when you first have the inclination or thought to do that activity.

At this point, notice without fixing, correcting, or putting yourself in what you think is the "right" posture to begin the action. Making an adjustment at this point may result in another layer of tightening and contraction on top of what may already be a tense situation.

Observations:
- Notice the moment you have the thought to do the activity. This may happen very quickly and it may take some time to identify when you have the first impulse to do something.
- Notice how quickly your mind and body jump in to accomplish the task.
- Notice if you stay physically conscious throughout the task.
- Where is your mind while you accomplish the task?

four: how to change your patterns

Your Moment of Awareness and Choice
Fig. 7 Balanced Posture

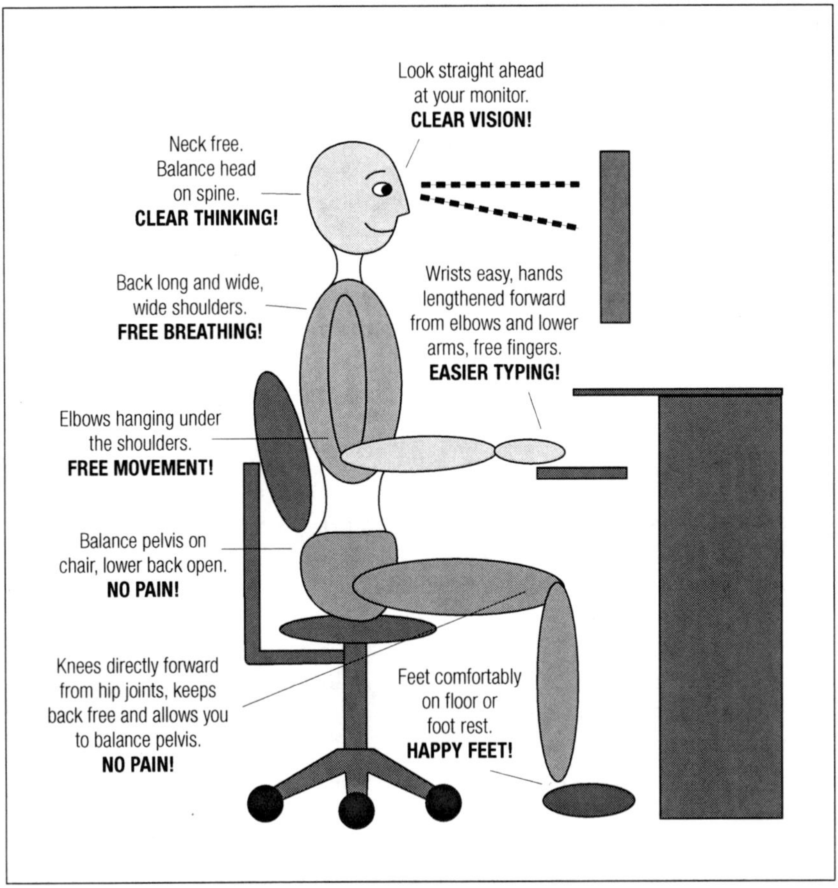

- Look straight ahead at your monitor. **CLEAR VISION!**
- Neck free. Balance head on spine. **CLEAR THINKING!**
- Back long and wide, wide shoulders. **FREE BREATHING!**
- Wrists easy, hands lengthened forward from elbows and lower arms, free fingers. **EASIER TYPING!**
- Elbows hanging under the shoulders. **FREE MOVEMENT!**
- Balance pelvis on chair, lower back open. **NO PAIN!**
- Knees directly forward from hip joints, keeps back free and allows you to balance pelvis. **NO PAIN!**
- Feet comfortably on floor or foot rest. **HAPPY FEET!**

Current Habits
- Past experience
- Idea of what is "right"
- What you already know
- Security
- I am going to "do" it
- In a rush

New Choice
- Allowing for less force
- Taking a chance
- New possibilities
- Less stress
- Staying centered
- Easier movement
- Clearer

Step 2: Alert Pause / Active Non-doing

The next step in consciously changing your movement pattern for the better is to actively pause. In other words, do not go on automatic pilot to do the task. This does not mean to freeze your actions in place and become a statue! Rather, simply take a brief moment to stop your normal response to the activity you are about to do. Sometimes it is useful to come to a total halt, but that is not necessarily desirable. It is important to learn to think while keeping the flow going. You are inhibiting your normal action and actively non-doing.

You will find a strong connection between the impulse to take action and the actual motion to perform the action with your body. Often the body is in motion even before the thought to act is becoming conscious. This is where your awareness has to become sharp and clear.

The task here is to stop your response BEFORE you make any muscular movement toward doing an activity. This is an interesting moment – not responding to the idea of doing something. Pay attention at a very subtle level to see how you respond to tasks you perform all the time. See if you can wait a moment (even while activity is continuing) before moving and responding.

Putting Step 1 and Step 2 together, use these activities to practice first identifying the impulse to do them and then very briefly actively pausing before you go into the action.

Good practice activities:
- Put your hands on the keyboard.
- Answer an urgent email.
- Stand up from your chair.

Notice the manner in which you want to respond and then ACTIVELY PAUSE.

Notice if there is a difference in your response to a stimulus you do by yourself and when other people are involved.

Step 3: Balance and Redirect Yourself / Make a Choice

If you have made any preparations to do the activity let those go in Step 3. Let go of any tensions that may have accumulated in the moments of identifying the stimulus and the active pause. This doesn't mean to collapse or shrink in any way. Release any extra tension that was accumulated in your response to the stimulus so you are allowing for new movement potential. You are establishing your best balance and sense of movement and energetic flow and direction.

As you drop any unnecessary tensions your natural body balance and flow of energy will emerge. Your structure and system have an innate lengthening and widening you can consciously perceive. By focusing on freeing your neck and allowing your head to lead your body gently in an upward direction you can enhance this sense of lengthening and widening of your body. You will experience your natural three-dimensionality and the rebound from gravity. This will affect your entire body.

From the active pause let go again. Let go of more and more tension that may have accumulated. Notice that you can consciously stay with the lengthening and widening. You will simultaneously sense more of your weight on the ground and an upward direction throughout your entire body. Again, this is not a passive releasing of the neck nor a reaching upwards but a palpable and strong sense of upward movement from the floor as you stay on the ground.

You may find yourself taking a spontaneous inhale as you stop fixing or setting yourself.

There can be a tendency to try too hard to stay long by reaching the head up away from the body. This actually diminishes the width of the body and takes away from the natural suspension system. Play with how easily you can balance your head on the top of your spine and the resultant sense of opening of the body and freedom of your movement.

As you stay with it, you learn not to respond to the stimulus in your usual way. You will have less and less tension to let go of. Steps 1-3 can happen very quickly. They don't have to take a lot of time. They do take attention and thought.

four: how to change your patterns

Thoughts to give yourself:
- Keep your neck free.
- Allow your head to balance and gently direct your whole head up at the top of your spine.
- Allow your back to follow the head creating lengthening and widening in the back and torso.
- Allow your entire body to follow the upward direction of your head while you sense your body weight on the chair.
- Let your legs be easy as you sit on your sit bones.

These directions will emerge naturally as you release the tensions in your body. This establishes a base of support and sense of motion in your body from which to move. It is important not to manufacture these directions and flow of energy by reaching up with your head or placing your body in a particular manner.

Step 4: Move With Ease / Response

Start your action from this new balanced and directed situation. Your directions are in place and working so you will be able to move without any preparation. Your movements will emerge from the balanced sense of movement flow that has come from letting go of unnecessary tensions.

Allow for unfamiliar sensations and new movements to occur. New ways of responding are going to create new sensations and ways of being.

Clues:
- Let your movement be light, easy, and fluid.
- Let your movement feel different than it normally does.
- Keep breathing.
- Letting go of any amount of excess tension is helpful.

Begin your movements:
- In a smooth manner without any suddenness or quick starts. This does not mean to go in slow motion but to allow the movement to emerge from the existing flow.
- Without any new unnecessary muscular tension.
- With as little force as possible.
- From the existing movement flow.

chapter five
Sample Activity – Answering the Phone

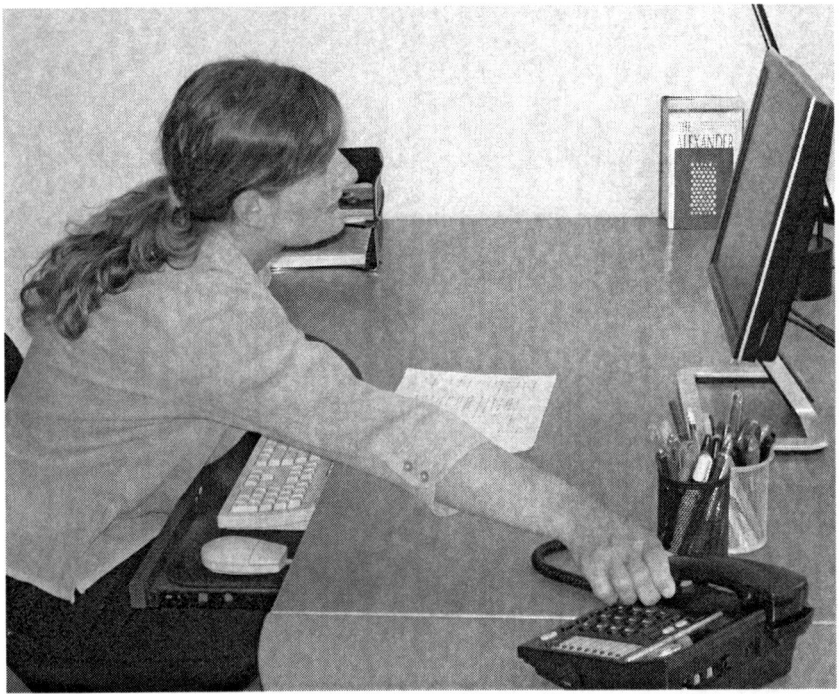

Fig. 8 Is this you?

Step 1: Observe What Happens When the Phone Rings

- Does your hand automatically reach for the phone as soon as you hear it ring?
- Do you anticipate who is on the other end?
- Do you clench your jaw?
- Do you stop breathing?
- Do you raise your shoulders?
- Fill in your own observations.

five: sample activity – answering the phone

Step 2: Active Pause

Allow yourself one more ring of the phone before you answer to give yourself time to inhibit your initial response.

- Stop yourself from carrying out your initial impulse.
- Notice what you want to do and don't do it.
- ACTIVELY PAUSE and wait a moment.

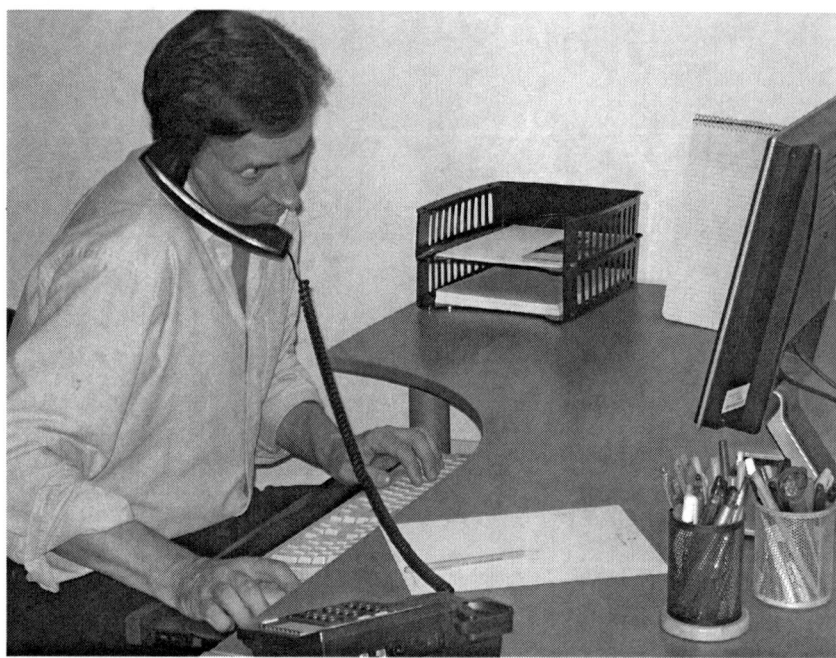

Fig. 9 Harmful phone posture

Step 3: Balance and Redirect Yourself

- Keep breathing.
- Let go of any tension in your neck.
- Let your head gently direct up away from your spine.
- Allow your weight to drop onto the chair.
- Keep your shoulder, elbow, wrist, and hand free of tension.
- Notice the upward direction that emerges in your body.

five: sample activity – answering the phone

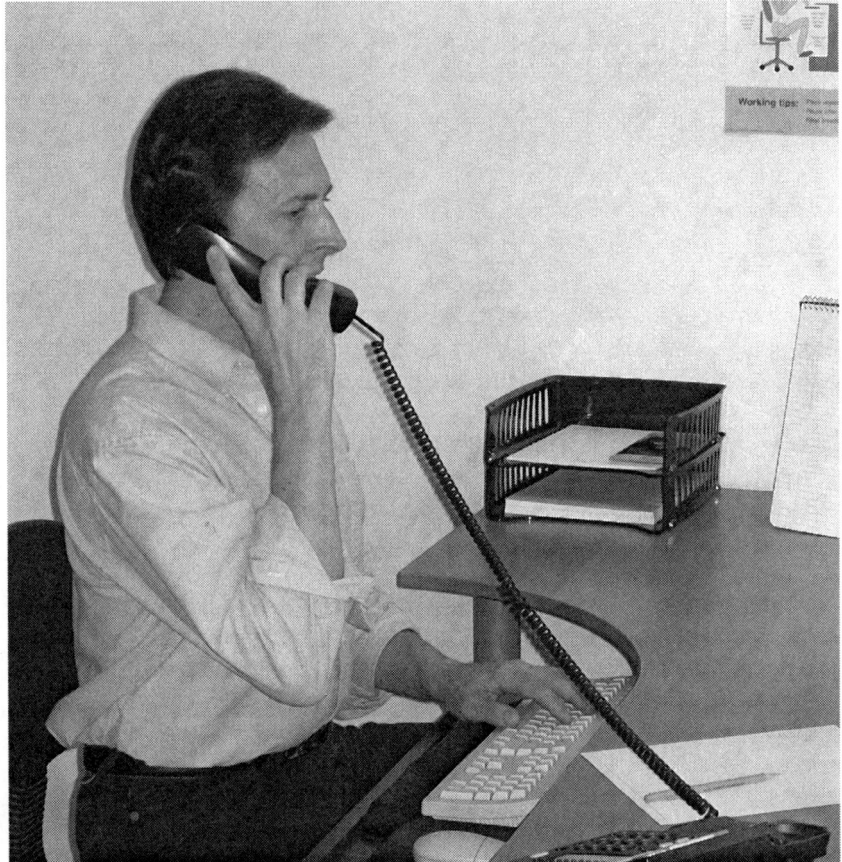

Fig. 10 Bring the phone to your head.

Step 4: Answer the Phone Easily and Without Expectations

- Hold the phone lightly – no gripping.
- Bring the phone up to your head rather than leaning your head forward to meet the phone.
- Take a breath in before you speak.
- Stay upright while you speak.
- Give the caller your full attention.

chapter six

Step 3 Expanded: What to Think and Notice

As you redirect your thoughts in Step 3 there are many ideas that will inform your awareness and thinking. Your body will respond to your thoughts even though you may not readily experience it. Your awareness will develop as you stick with the thought processes.

Direct yourself gently. It is important not to jerk your body, hold, or place yourself in a new position. This may just layer on new tensions and habits over the already existing habits. The goal is to undo your unproductive habits so you move in the most naturally balanced way possible.

As you understand how to direct yourself you will realize there is the potential for movement all the time. You are a moving body even when you think you are still. You may describe this movement potential as being:

- Loose
- Easy
- Ready to move
- Free in the joints
- Light
- Open

The following are some specific ideas worth thinking about. They are all aspects of the same goal – an integrated mind-body.

Starting at the Top: Head and Neck

How your head balances and is directed on your spine are key in your overall functioning. Your head leads your body and your body follows.

When your head is freely poised at the top of your spine the downward pressure many of us put on ourselves is released and a lengthening and widening of the torso is triggered. Taking this pressure off the body (the head weighs 10-12 pounds!) helps reduce backache, poor breathing, neck pain, and so on.

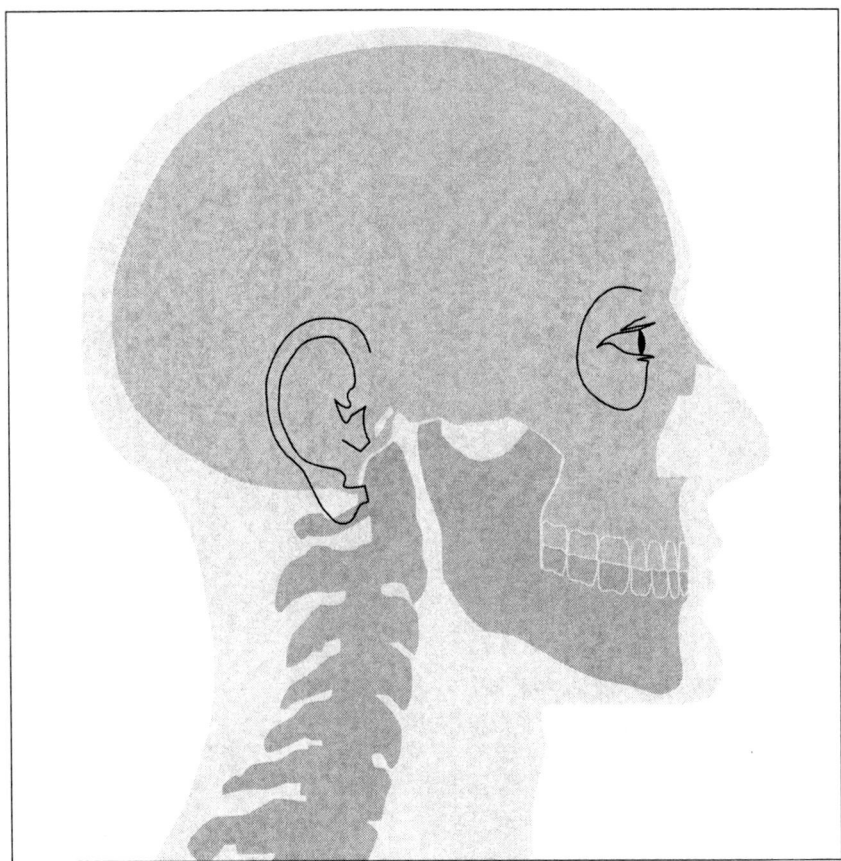

Fig. 11 How the head and neck relate

Notice in Fig. 11 and experience in your body that:
- You have head both in front of and behind the point of balance.
- Your neck comes up behind your jaw – all the way up behind your nose.
- You have a lot of head above your eyes.
- Your neck has a natural curve.
- Your head has a lot of depth (front to back space).

six: step 3 expanded: what to think and notice

Thoughts to give yourself:
- Allow your head to balance and be free at the top of your spine (There is no need to hold your head onto your neck).
- Gently allow your head to direct up off your spine (no reaching or pulling).
- When looking down, bend from the top of your spine while keeping your whole spine lengthened.
- Move from the top of your spine (behind your nose) when looking to the side.

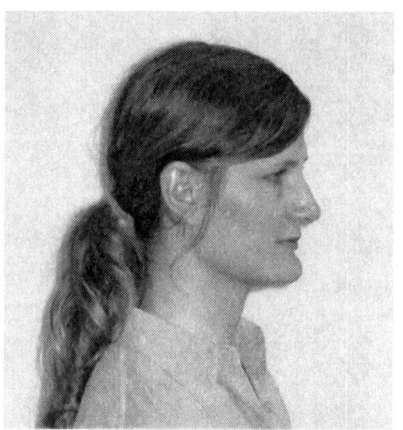

Fig. 12 Good balance of head on spine

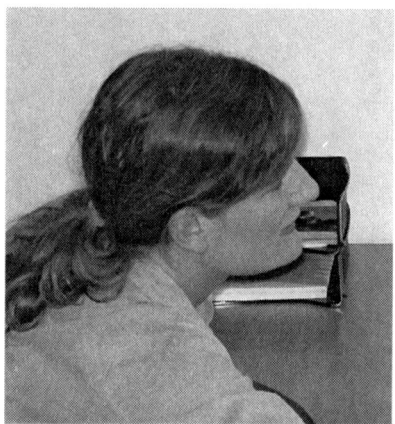

Fig. 13 Shortened neck, pulling head off balance

Practice Activity – Saying "Yes" and "No"

Practice identifying where your head and neck meet by nodding "yes" from the top of your spine. Move from the same high place when you nod "no."

Each time you are about to nod your head, stop for a moment, let your neck go, and then nod "yes" or "no."

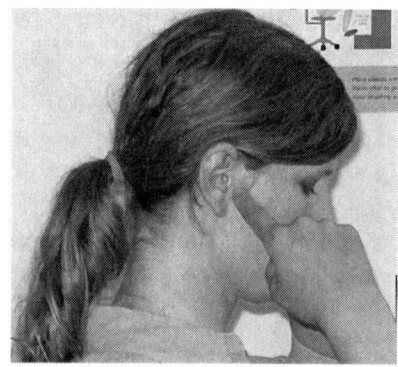

Fig. 14 Head nods "yes" on the axis between your ears

six: step 3 expanded: what to think and notice

How You See: Eyes

Your eyes lead your head. Where and how you look and see affect your face and entire body. The way we use our eyes is as habitual as the way we use any part of the body.

Your eyeballs themselves only receive light and information. They are the sensory receptors, not the interpreters, of information. The part of your brain, the visual cortex, that makes sense of the light that your eyes receive is in the back of your head.

If you find yourself squinting your eyes or narrowing your face, make sure the lighting in your workspace is adequate. There should be no glare on your screen or lights shining directly into your eyes.

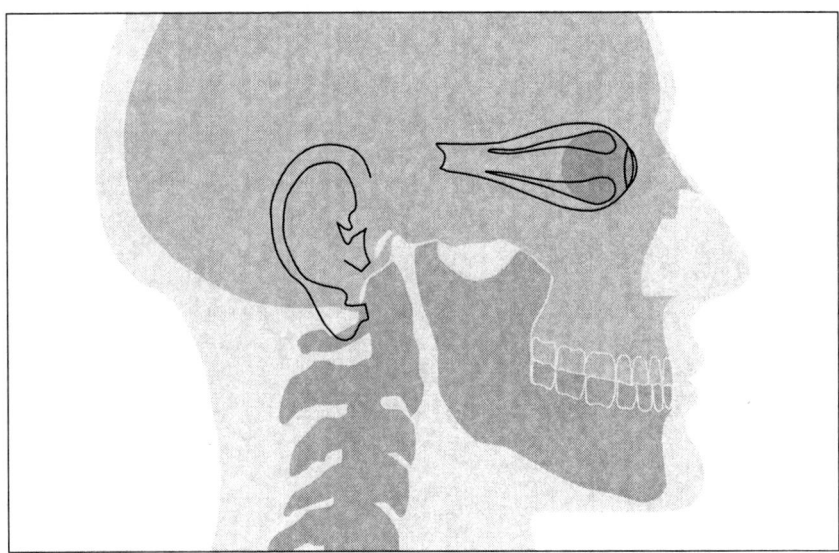

Fig. 15 Depth of eye socket

Notice in Fig. 15 and experience in your body:
- The depth of your eye socket: how far back into your skull your eyes go.
- The shape of your eyeballs: they are three-dimensional.

Notice how you use your eyes when you are very focused on a topic, learning something new, or trying to remember something from the past.

30

six: step 3 expanded: what to think and notice

Thoughts to give yourself for using your eyes in an easy and relaxed way:
- Allow the images and light from your computer or paper to come into your eyes.
- Include the use of your peripheral vision. When you look at your computer, see the room around you outside the computer screen.
- Look away from your workstation frequently. This will help you rest your eyes.
- Close or cover your eyes with your hands to block out all the surrounding light for a few moments and consciously let go of your eye muscles. This is known as "palming."
- Inscribe very large circles in space with your eye focus (not your whole head), looking both clockwise and counterclockwise. Make sure you draw complete circles.

Practice Activity – Looking at an Object
Pick one activity you do frequently such as looking at your computer screen, glancing at your keyboard, or looking at your calendar. As you move your gaze to that object, consciously let your eyes relax and soften while you take in and see that object. Consciously see that object while at the same time seeing the peripheral space around the object. Stay with that expanded focus as long as your vision is on the object. With practice, including your peripheral vision will not distract you from the specific object you are looking at. In fact, you will begin to see more and more clearly, from specific details to the big picture.

Jaw and Tongue

The tongue and jaw are areas where many of us hold stress and tension. When they let go, it helps to free the neck, balance the head on the spine, and breathe better.

The movement of the jaw and tongue can be done without disturbing the balance of the head on the spine, because your jaw moves in relation to the skull. The jawbone does not attach to the bones of the neck.

Notice in Fig. 16 and experience in your body that:
- The jaw joint is back by the ears.
- There is quite a bit of space between the lower jaw and the neck.
- The teeth end before the back of the jaw. In other words, there is more jaw bone behind your back teeth. The teeth don't continue to the back of the jaw near your neck.

six: step 3 expanded: what to think and notice

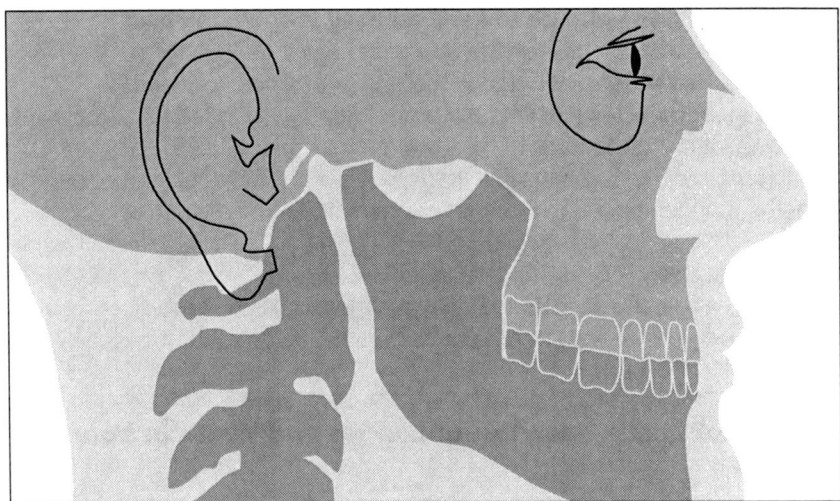

Fig. 16 Jaw on skull

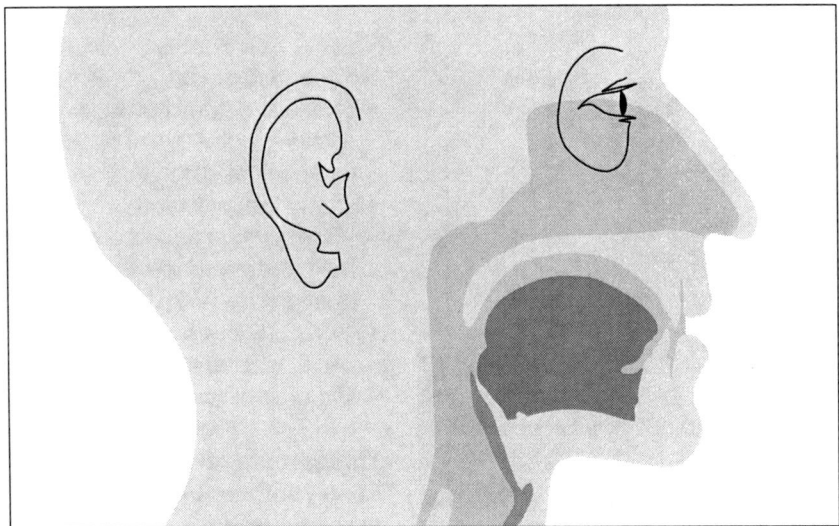

Fig. 17 Cross section of the tongue and jaw

Notice in Fig. 17 and experience in your body:
- The size of the tongue – large!
- The middle and back of the tongue can be up fairly high in the mouth.
- Your tongue and jaw can move independently from one another.

32

six: step 3 expanded: what to think and notice

Thoughts to give yourself to keep an easy tongue and jaw:
- Keep a little space between the upper and lower teeth.
- Keep the jaw in the joint and don't let the jaw be heavy or passive.
- Allow the tongue to sit high in the mouth with the rounded tip of the tongue touching the back of the lower teeth.
- Keep the tongue free and wide (it might touch the sides of your upper teeth). It doesn't need to push up or down while you are at rest.

Practice Activity – Breathing
As you exhale keep a little space between the upper and lower teeth. Let the air move up over the top of your tongue as you breathe out.

Your Head Leads Your Torso: Length and Width of Your Back

As your head gently moves up off your spine you will sense an energy and movement flow up through your body. This is the primary support system for all of your movement.

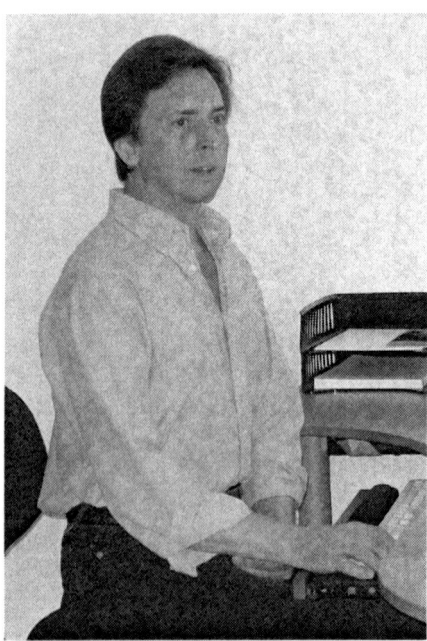

Fig. 18 Long and easy head/neck/torso

Notice in Fig. 18:
- You have natural curves in your spine – part of their function is for shock absorption.
- Your whole torso and back include both your chest and pelvis.
- The back of your pelvis is included in the width of your back.
- As you stay with your back, this will support and free your ribs and breathing.

Thoughts to give yourself to keep your back long, wide, and pain free:
- Allow your torso to follow the upward direction of your head without pushing or pulling yourself upward.
- Keep your back in the back part of your body.

six: step 3 expanded: what to think and notice

- Remember your spine is in the back and middle part of your torso.

Practice Activity – Head Leading

Take a walk around your office area and down the hall. Allow your neck to be free and your head to gently direct. Notice how this takes weight off your body and gives you an overall sense of lightness. You might notice that your overall gait is lighter and you are making less sound on the floor.

Ongoing Motion: Breathing

As you observe your breathing you will notice that it is an essential aspect of keeping your natural flow and balance and movement potential.

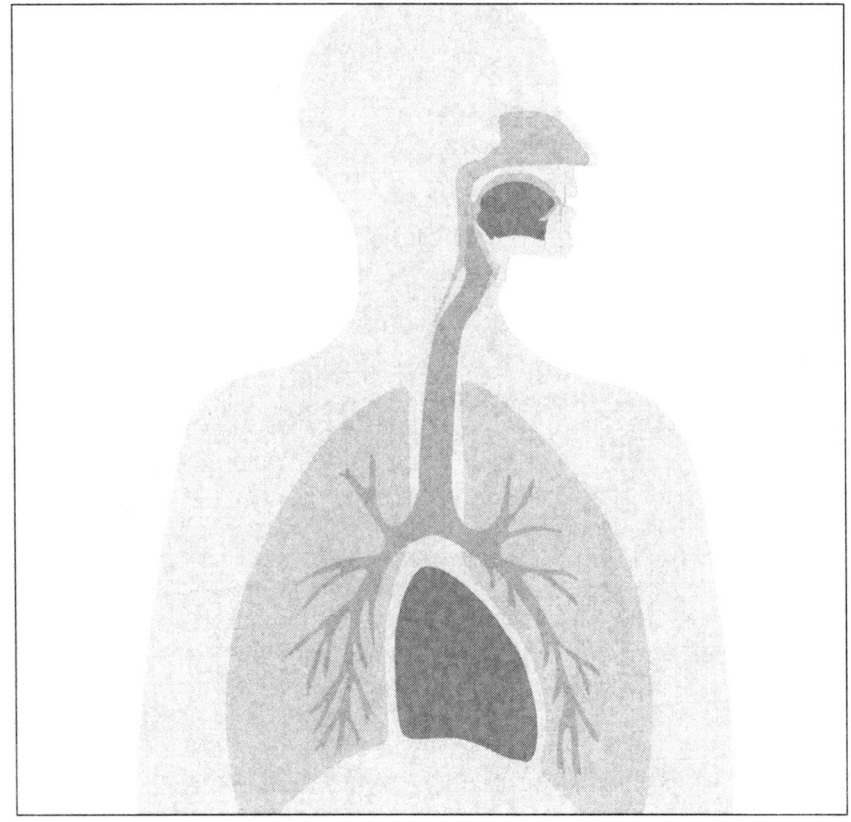

Fig. 19 Side view of head, front view of chest

six: step 3 expanded: what to think and notice

Notice in Fig. 19 and experience in your body:
- How long your air passage is.
- That your lungs surround your heart.
- How much more air space there is at the bottom of your lungs than the top.

Also notice:
- What stimuli cause you to diminish or stop breathing and hold your breath.
- How you can sense your weight on the chair more easily while you are breathing easily.
- Allow the breath to come in and out freely. Don't suck or pull the air in or push the air out.
- Your neck, shoulders, and entire body soften when you are breathing easily.

Thoughts to give yourself:
- When you find you haven't been breathing, let air out first before you inhale.
- Allow the air to come into your body easily.
- Allow your ribs to move and respond to the internal movement of the air.

Practice Activity – Continuous Breathing
Notice if and when you stop your breathing. Check that you are breathing when you pick up the phone, listen to your boss or colleague, type at your computer, and walk to the water cooler.

Connect to the Chair: Pelvis

Your pelvis balances on the chair (and on your legs when standing) like your head balances on your spine. Freedom in the legs and pelvis while you are sitting allows you to maintain a dynamic support for your back, shoulders, arms, and hands. It allows you to release your legs and actually let the chair support your body weight.

Notice in Fig. 20 and experience in your body that:
- Your hip joints are below the crest of your pelvis.
- Your pelvis has an up and down dimension.
- Your sit bones are below your thighbones.
- Your thighbones aren't touching the chair.
- The hip joints themselves are closer to your midline than to the bone at the outside of your upper leg.

six: step 3 expanded: what to think and notice

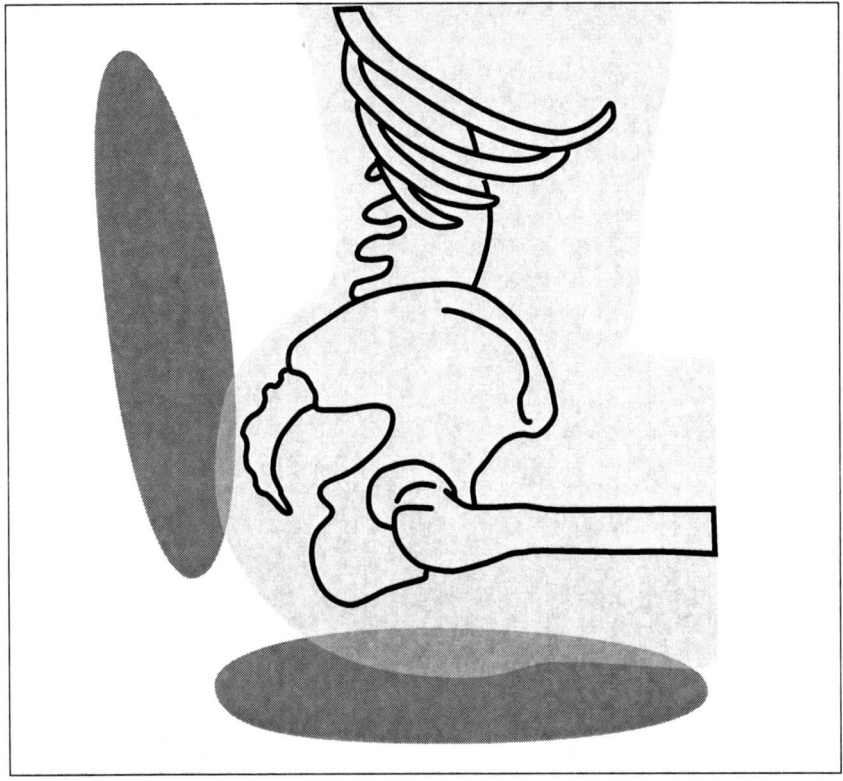

Fig. 20 Pelvis on the chair

Thoughts to give yourself as you sit on the chair:
- Allow the weight of your torso to flow through your pelvis into your sit bones and onto the chair (making sure you don't collapse).
- Let your pelvis move with the rest of your torso in following the upward direction of your head.
- When you tilt forward to reach for something or to stand, rock forward on your sit bones.

Practice Activity – Defining the Whole Torso
Keeping your back long and wide, tilt forward in your chair. Let your head lead and your body follow as you rock forward on your sit bones. This action will increase the crease and fold in your hip joint. This is a good activity to perform when your back hurts, you feel fatigue, or you feel you need a break but you can't leave your desk.

Connect to the Floor: Legs and Feet

Allow yourself to sit on the chair. That means you can let your body weight go into the chair (again, that doesn't mean to sink or collapse). Although you are not directly standing on your feet they do provide a reference for your legs and back. Thus they help you balance and give you stability while you sit. Leaving your legs alone, not holding on or overusing them while sitting, keeps the legs from pulling or pushing on the back. That in turn allows your back to work with more ease, frees up your breathing, and lets you lengthen and widen your entire back from your sit bones on up through your body.

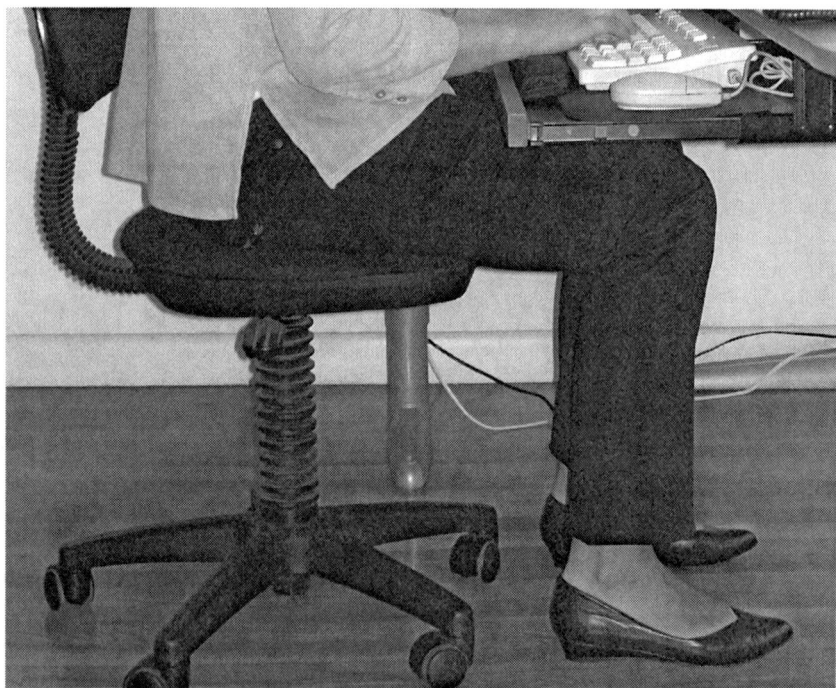

Fig. 21 Knees forward from the hips and feet flat on the floor

Notice in Fig. 21 and experience in your body that:
- Your sit bones are on the seat of the chair.
- There is a difference between your legs and your pelvis.
- Your legs are in front of your back and your back is behind your legs.

six: step 3 expanded: what to think and notice

Thoughts to give yourself to connect to the floor:
- Your thighs rest.
- Keep in mind the whole leg: upper side, middle where the bone is, and under side that is in contact with the chair.
- Allow your knees to lead your thigh forward from your hip joints.
- Keep a bit of space between your knees so they are going away from each other.
- Let your feet connect with the floor below your knees.
- Allow your feet to spread out on the floor.

Practice Activity – What Is the Torso and What Are the Legs
Let your knees rock forward and way from each other while you leave your torso long. Stay long out your head. You can move your legs in and out without disturbing the balance and length of your torso, head, and neck.

Lift one knee, and thus the entire leg, so your entire leg is up off the seat of the chair and set it back down again without disturbing the balance of your torso, head, and neck. Connect the non-moving leg into the floor for support. This activity takes skill and a long back.

Typing: Arms, Wrists, and Hands

How you use your arms and hands in relation to your back while working at your desk is paramount. When your back is long and wide, your arms and hands move freely in your joints and extend from your back.

Notice in Fig. 22 and experience in your body:
- The shoulder joints are out at the sides of your body.
- There is space between your arms and your chest at the sides of your body.
- The lower arm has two bones in it allowing for rotation toward the thumb side of the lower arm. This means you can rotate the lower arm a good amount without the shoulder moving. (This rotation is what allows your palms to face your keyboard without your shoulders coming forward).
- There are many bones in the hand between the wrist and the fingers. These bones allow for moving the fingers without disturbing the rest of the arm.

six: step 3 expanded: what to think and notice

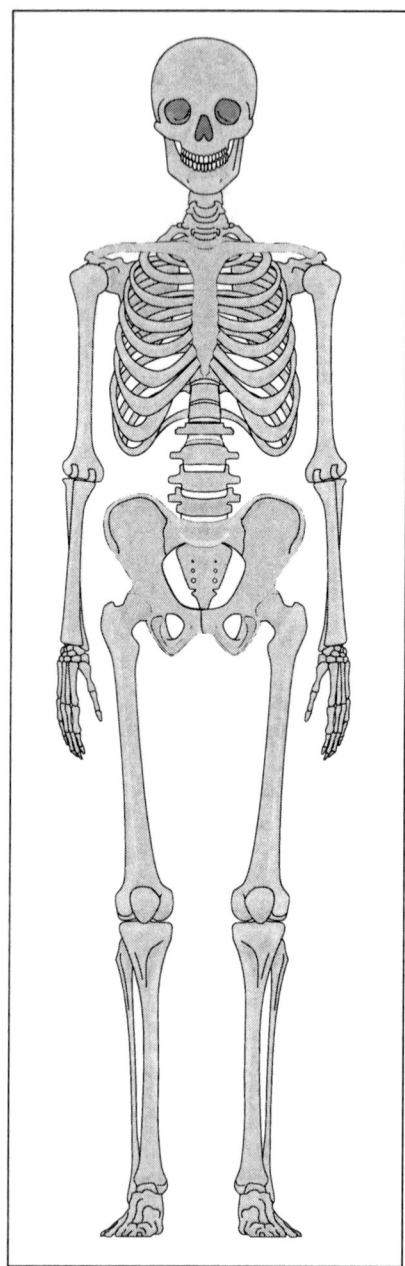

Fig 22 Skeleton viewed from the front

Notice in Fig. 23 and experience in your body:
- The shoulder, elbows, and wrists are movable and can adapt to the necessary movement. Your joints bend when you reach for objects near you.
- The wrists are slightly below the elbows.
- The elbows are slightly in front of the shoulders.
- There is plenty of room to move the arms and hands in the workspace.
- There is no leaning onto the keyboard. The back is supporting the arms.
- The angle of the wrists while typing.
- The curve in the fingers.
- The fingers are soft and fluid.

Thoughts to give yourself:
- Keep breathing while you are thinking and typing.
- Let the width of your back continue out to your elbows.
- Let your hands be in front and away from your back and, conversely, your back be behind your hands.
- Allow your thumbs to be easy, not hyper-extended or tucked under the palm.
- Keep your shoulders with your torso.
- Allow your hands to be a continuation of your forearms.
- Let your fingers curve forward and away from your palm.
- Widen the palm of your hand.

six: step 3 expanded: what to think and notice

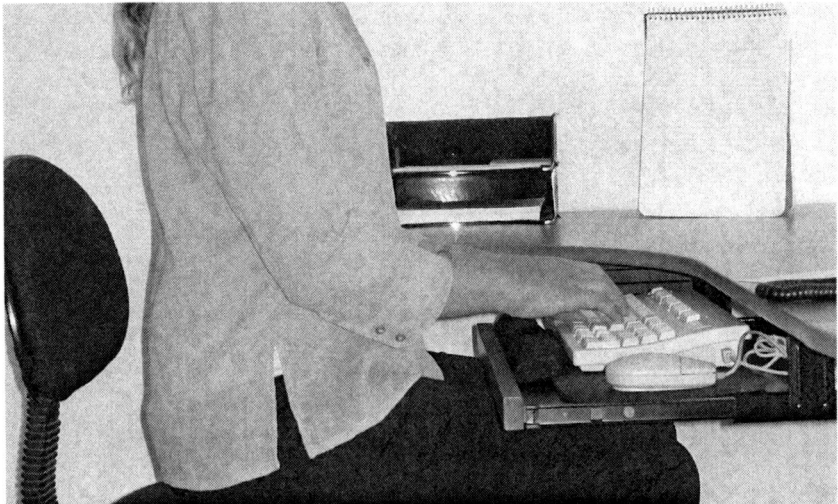

Fig. 23 Good relationship of arms to the keyboard

- Lengthen your fingertips away from your shoulders through your elbows and wrists.
- Keep the weight of your arms off the keyboard so you are not leaning on the keys or computer in any way.

Practice Activity 1: Moving the Lower Arm – Radial Rotation
Place your lower arm on the desk, resting on the little finger side with the thumb side going up toward the ceiling. Keeping the little finger side of the lower arm and the elbow in place on the table, allow the thumb side of the hand to drop toward the table so the palm is facing down on the table. Then rotate the lower arm (still keeping the little finger side of the lower arm on the table) so the back of the hand is on the table. Rotate the lower arm around the little finger side of the lower arm several times (radial rotation).

You will notice that there is quite a lot of movement in the lower arm that can occur without the movement of the upper arm. Each of us has our own range of motion so the amount of movement will differ from person to person; however, most people discover more movement than they thought possible when performing this activity.

This is also a helpful activity to do if your wrist is tight or uncomfortable.

40

Practice Activity 2 – Preparing to Type

Each time you bring your hands to the keyboard become aware of the movement that is happening in your arms and upper body. As you keep your back long and wide you will be able to bring your hands (through bending your elbows) up to the keyboard without lowering your shoulders or bringing them forward.

Remember the width of your back continues out to your elbows.

Practice Activity 3 – Loose Wrists and Hands

Play around with typing while keeping your arms loose and free as you strike the keys (keep your body weight on the chair). Think of the energy in your arm subtly going through your wrist into the keyboard as though you are casting spells into the keyboard with each keystroke.

Words on the Screen: Pressure / Force on the Keyboard

It is possible to let your fingers fly on the keyboard. In order to allow your thoughts to flow easily onto the page it is necessary to lighten your touch and allow your movements to be as easy and free as possible. It may feel out of control when you start to let up on the force you are using. The more you work with a lighter touch on the keyboard, the faster you will become.

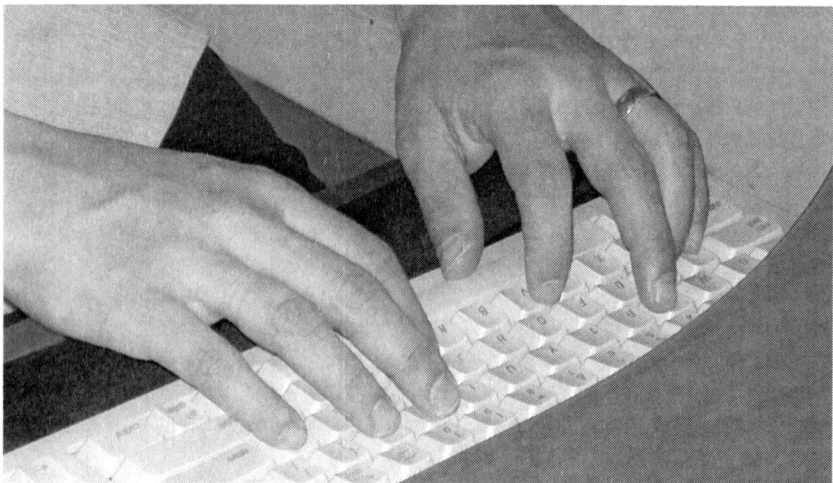

Fig. 24 Easy wrists, hands, and fingers

six: step 3 expanded: what to think and notice

Notice as you type:
- What parts of your arm-wrist-hand-fingers are being used to strike each key.
- The amount of force you are using to strike your keyboard.
- Your body weight on the chair while you are typing.

Thoughts to give yourself:
- Leave your shoulders alone while you are typing.
- Use only the tips of your fingers to strike the keys on your keyboard.
- Sense your fingertips contacting the keyboard.
- Keep breathing.

Practice Activity – Minimal Force
Take a few minutes to experiment with your keyboard to see how much pressure is really needed to get the letters to appear on the screen. The first step is to make contact with the keys by touching them and then start the pressure to see how much force it takes to get the letter to show up on the screen. Play with each finger to see if you use more pressure with one finger than another. Treat this like a game. Then speed up your typing and maintain your easy typing, using only as much force as necessary. Imagine that you are playing the piano as you type and you are playing at a very soft volume so you don't have to use much force to create sound.

Notice that your arms and hands are working less when you use less force. You will probably be able to type more quickly and accurately as you type with more ease.

Mousing Around: Hands and Mouse

Find a mouse that feels comfortable in your hand. Some people like their whole palm to connect with the mouse while others prefer to move just their fingers. Whatever you choose, make sure you put your mouse within easy reach.

Notice:
- What you do with your neck when you reach for your mouse.
- How much pressure you use while contacting your mouse.
- How much force and pressure you use to move your mouse around.
- What part of your hand you use to move your mouse.

six: step 3 expanded: what to think and notice

Thoughts to give yourself:
- When reaching for your mouse, allow your elbow to extend.
- Sense the volume of the mouse in your palm.
- Grasp the mouse very lightly.
- Move the mouse from your fingertips.
- Sense the mouse moving on the horizontal plane.

Practice Activity – Light Touch
Play around with how easily you can contact and touch your mouse, much as you did with how you made contact with the keyboard. See how easily you can move the mouse around without any particular destination on the screen. Then start to direct the mouse toward a particular point and maintain that ease of movement.

chapter seven
Working at a Laptop Computer

Many people work at laptop computers. The convenience of having a portable computer is wonderful, and it also has its hazards.

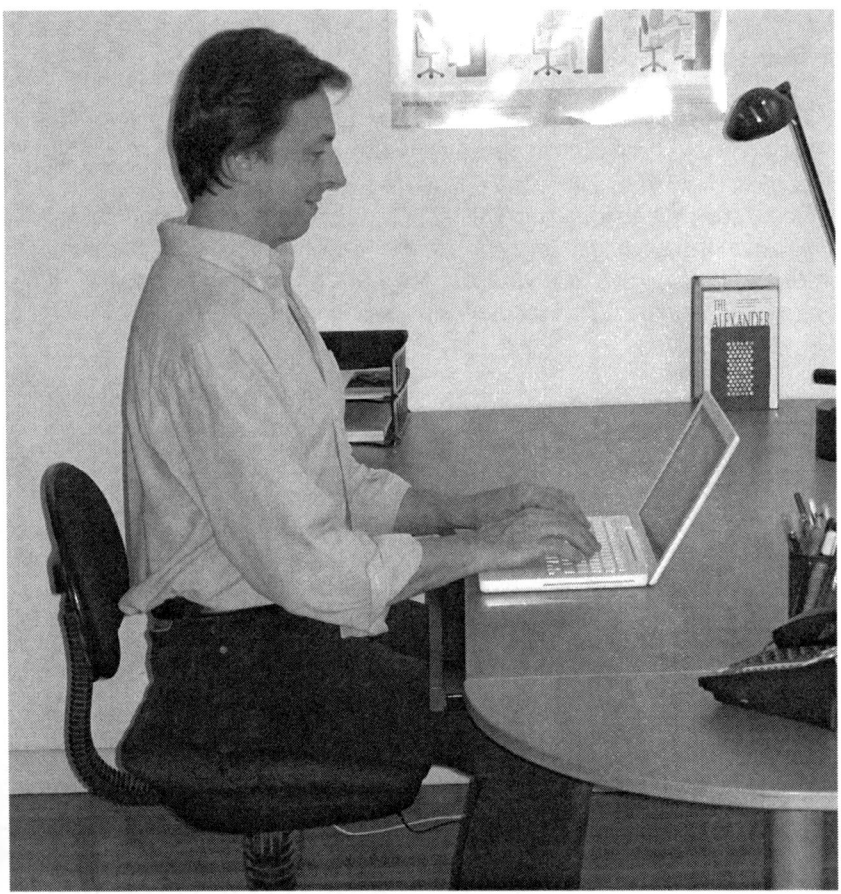

Fig. 25 Working with a laptop

seven: working at a laptop computer

It is recommended that at your most permanent laptop workstation you obtain an external monitor and/or keyboard. This allows you to separate the keyboard from the screen and adjust the workstation to fit your body proportions.

A separate keyboard can be obtained for a relatively small amount of money. It is well worth the investment.

As often as possible, sit at a desk or table to work at your laptop. That way you can minimize the variables and find your best balance.

When you are traveling or taking your laptop to a meeting or the couch there are several things you can do to work with more ease:
- Tilt the screen so you can see it easily.
- Find a place where there is no glare on the screen.
- Tilt your head from the top of your spine as you look at the screen. This will keep you from putting stress on your back and neck.
- Look up frequently (more than usual) to rest your eyes and back.
- Resist the urge to lounge on the couch with your laptop. Often in this situation the back is tilted back and the neck becomes tight in the front.
- When the computer is in your lap, put a pillow underneath it so the screen is higher and your lower arms are horizontal.

chapter eight
Working on the Bed

Many people who work at home use their bed as both a chair and a desk. If this is the arrangement you have set up supply yourself with enough pillows and flat writing surfaces to create a situation with different levels on your bed.

As much as possible, find a physical setup that allows you to meet the best balance ideas presented in Chapter 3.

These ideas can also be used by people who like to work while sitting on the floor. The floor may be more adaptable as there are low coffee tables that can easily serve as a desk surface.

Warning: When you are sitting well in a chair at your desk your back strengthens itself through good use. One of the consequences of working on a bed, is that people often lean against pillows and allow the back to curve in a "C" shape. This posture does not naturally strengthen the back through use as it is not really being used. The pillows are doing the support that the muscles are meant to do. This can lead to a weak back that is prone to aches and pains.

Include in your setup:
- Support for your back so your back can be long and vertical. This will keep pressure off the front of your neck.
- Find a way to allow for bending in your hips, knees, and ankles.
- Prop up your computer so you can see the screen easily. If you put a laptop on your knees or thighs, elevate it with a pillow so you can see the screen easily. There will probably have to be a compromise between the screen height (affecting your neck) and the angle of your arms (affecting your shoulders, arms, wrists, and hands).
- A clear pathway so you can get up and walk around frequently.
- Keep papers, writing implements, and resource books close at hand.

chapter nine
Writing with Pen and Paper

Although most of us spend the majority of our time on the computer while sitting at our desks, there are still moments when we use a pen or pencil and paper.

Here are some important hints for using a pen and paper:
- Look down at the paper from the top of your spine so your back can remain long and wide.
- Maintain the width of your back and allow that width out through both elbows. No matter how wide your back is structurally, sensing and allowing for width of your back is key.
- Choose a pen that glides easily across the page so you don't have to press down into the paper to make a mark on the page.
- Hold the pen as lightly as possible.
- Keep your forearm easy as you write, allowing your fingers to do the moving.
- Consciously write along the horizontal surface of the paper.
- When moving your hand across the page, move from your elbow.
- Allow the words from the page to come up into your eyes so you can keep your eyes soft.
- Notice the white space on the page around the black letters and words

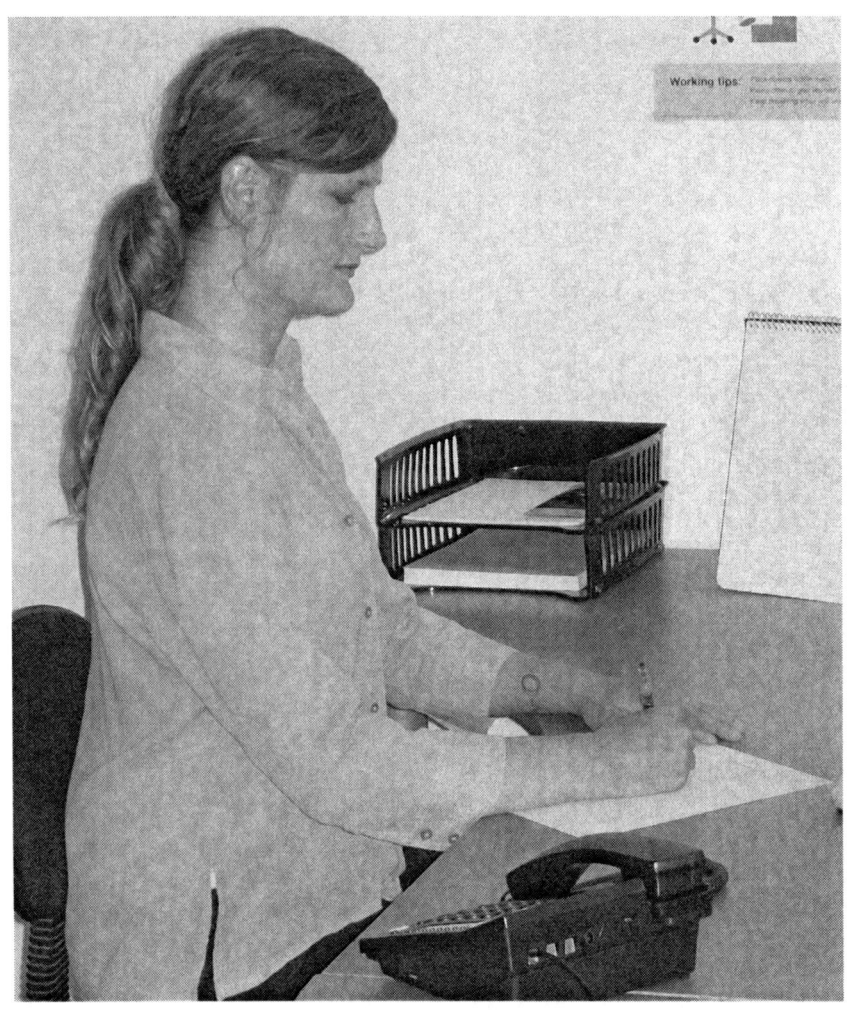

Fig. 26 Stay long and wide while you write with pen and paper

chapter ten
What to Think When...

Thinking of the following ideas is enough to break your pattern of stress and tension. The mind/body are so intimately connected that even a small thought will help break your pattern. If you practice "thinking" rather than "doing" you won't layer another habit on top of what is already there. Through thinking you will undo the habit you have going on and help yourself find your natural sense of balance and ease within your body.

Your Back Aches:
- Find your head on top of your spine.
- Keep your neck easy and free.
- Sense your weight on the chair.
- Lean forward and back a few times folding in your hip joints.
- Lengthen your back starting with the top of your head.
- Allow yourself to have the natural curves in your back.
- Keep breathing.

Your Neck Hurts:
- Think of your whole neck releasing.
- Make sure you are not holding your head on your spine.
- Allow for the natural curve in your neck and upper and lower parts of your back.
- Move your head from the top of your spine.
- Allow your tongue to be easy and wide.
- Release your jaw. Find space between your upper and lower teeth.

Your Shoulders Ache:
- Sense the width across your shoulders and back.
- Sense the width of your back out to your elbows.
- Sense the width of the front of your chest.
- Make sure you are not pinching your shoulder blades together.
- Keep your head over your chest and pelvis.
- Allow your weight to drop into your chair.
- Breathe into your width, especially up under your armpits.

Your Eyes Are Tired:
- Look up from your work.
- Look at an object in the distance.
- Let the muscles around your eyes release and soften.
- Close your eyes for a few minutes and then resume your work.
- Make sure there is no glare or light entering your eyes.
- Remember to allow the light from your work to come toward you.
- Palm your eyes (cover your eyes with your palms, blocking out all the light) to relieve tension.

Your Wrists and Hands Are Sore:
- Ease your neck and shoulders.
- Use less force on the keyboard.
- Put your hands in your lap and bring your hands up to your keyboard again with more ease, hands leading, elbows bending.
- Stretch your hands, wrists, forearms, and shoulders.

Your Feet Hurt:
- Allow your feet to spread out in your shoes.
- Stay easy in your ankles.
- Sense space between your toes.
- Let your heels release back onto the floor.

You Can't Think Anymore:
- Sense your weight on your chair.
- Think that you have an empty hollow head.
- Look up from your work.
- Close your eyes for a few moments.
- Roll your whole body forward sequentially, head leading, until the top of your head is pointing toward the floor. Roll back up to the vertical and resume your work.
- Walk to the rest room or drinking fountain.
- Bounce up and down or jump if you have the space and privacy.
- Make sure your breathing is continuous.

chapter eleven
Recuperation on the Job

Breaks help both your body and your mental focus. Flexibility in your body and mind are intertwined. Taking a break will allow you to work with more ease, focus, and efficiency.

There are times to keep plugging along when you are on a roll, and there are times when standing and stretching will allow you to renew your energy and come up with new ideas. Discover what works best for you. It is better to take a break BEFORE you feel the signs of stress or strain.

Build in recuperation times during your day that you can count on and look forward to. For instance, make sure you take a real lunch break. Eat at a location different from your workspace even if it is a table nearby.

Warning Signs that You Need a Break:
- Energy is low.
- Eyes hurt or are tired.
- Back, neck, arms, wrists, or shoulders ache.
- Breathing is shallow.
- Thinking and focus are fuzzy.
- Frustration level is high.
- Communications show agitation.
- Stomach is growling from hunger.

Short Breaks:
- Start over with your balanced sitting. Take your hands off the keyboard, put them in your lap, wait a moment while you breathe and find a better sitting balance, and place them with new awareness back on the keyboard.
- Exhale while you keep your length, an easy neck, tongue, and jaw, and allow the air to spring back into your body. Repeat 3 – 5 times.
- Close your eyes and allow your weight to drop into your chair. Give yourself 10 – 30 seconds with your eyes closed. Let your eyes rest back into your eye sockets.

- Look up away from your computer.
- Stand up and walk around your chair and then sit down.
- Stand up and balance on one leg – then on the other leg.
- Walk to the water cooler or rest room.
- Move your spine, led by your eyes, to curl down and arch up, twist right and left, bend side to side.
- Take your arms up above your head.
- Jump 10 – 15 times on a mini-trampoline of jump-rope (If that's possible).
- Drink water.

Longer Breaks:
- Take a walk outside to get a change of air, rest your eyes, and move your legs.
- Stand and stretch behind your chair or in a corner of the office.
- Make a quick personal phone call.
- Lie on your back for 10 – 15 minutes (if space and privacy are available).
- Meditate in your chair for 10 – 20 minutes.
- Take a lunchtime exercise or recuperation class.
- Visit a colleague for a few minutes.
- Take an extended coffee break.

chapter twelve
Getting to Work

You will also sit on the way to and from work in a car, on the bus, train, or subway. Although you aren't typing, writing, reading, or otherwise working, all of the sitting ideas you have learned so far apply.

Or you may have the good fortune to be able to walk to work. When this is possible, it is a great way to get some exercise and allow you to arrive at work energized and ready to go. Walking home after work is an opportunity to refresh and get ready for the rest of your day.

Here are some things to think about as you organize your travel time to support your time at work.

Sitting in the Car
- Take the time to readjust the driver's seat for your own body proportions. Do this every time you get into the car if you share it with other drivers. Adjust the seat height and distance from the steering wheel and pedals first so you are sitting at your full height. Then adjust the mirror.
- Add a pillow behind your back if needed so you can sit up vertically.
- Add a pillow under your pelvis to make the seat horizontal if it slants backward from your knees.
- Grasp the wheel firmly but without excess tension.
- Wear shoes that allow you to work the pedals of the car safely and easily.

Sitting on the Bus, Train, or Subway
- If the seats are curved or are "bucket" seats, it sometimes helps to sit at the front edge of the seat so you don't slump.
- If your ride is short and you will be sitting all day, consider standing during the ride.
- Spend some time taking a long view to encourage your eyes to change focus and relax.

Walking to Work
Walking deserves a more thorough discussion, but here are a few general concepts:
- Give yourself enough time to walk well and at a good pace without having to rush.
- Wear shoes that are comfortable, give support and cushioning, and allow you to move your ankles.
- Keep your head and neck easy the way you do while you are sitting.
- Allow your body to follow your head in an upward direction.
- When possible, let your arms swing easily back and forth in opposition to your legs as you walk.
- Look up at the space in front of you as you walk. Notice the ground about 15 – 20 feet out in front of you so you can keep a long view with your focus.
- Spend some time looking around to allow your eyes to relax and change focus as you enjoy your walk.

chapter thirteen
The Alexander Technique

Now that you have been working with the principles of the Alexander Technique, here is more theory and language to go with what you have been learning.

The Alexander Technique is a learning method for building awareness of how your mind and body are intimately related. It helps you discover how your thinking and moving connect and how you can consciously direct yourself into more optimal functioning. Through the Technique you will discover and refine fundamental movements that affect every movement you do in and out of the office.

The Technique is most often taught in a one-on-one setting where the student receives individual hands-on guidance in finding the best balance and use of the body.

One takes lessons to learn how to work on oneself much as you have been doing with the ideas and activities you have learned and explored in this book. The teacher can guide you to experience movement that is easier and freer.

In general we do what is familiar and sometimes we don't choose what is better and more balanced because it feels "wrong." It can be very useful, therefore, to have someone experienced in looking at habits lead you to new experiences.

As you have also learned from this book, the way you think about how you move and work makes a difference in the outcome of your movement and productivity. The Alexander teacher will help you uncover what you have been thinking in relation to how you have been moving and working.

The teacher will look at your whole body balance in relation to your activities. You will receive instruction that applies to all of your movement.

Often the private lesson will use the activity of getting in and out of a chair as a laboratory for the rest of your movement. It is a good time to learn how to keep your directions going while you start an activity and transfer your weight from your torso to your feet.

Private lessons may also include a time where you lie down on a table. In this situation you are invited to actively follow the teacher's hands while they help you experience how you can move without balancing your weight on your own feet. When you get up you will experience a greater lengthening and widening than you might find on your own. This helps you find new choices and expands your subtle movement vocabulary.

See the resources in Chapter 16 for how to find an Alexander Technique teacher in your area.

chapter fourteen
Review / Ideas To Remember

Here are some valuable tips to remember:

- You can expand your awareness to include your whole self while working.

- This is not about "sitting up straight."

- You are not working to find and hold the perfect "position."

- You are moving even when you think you are still.

- You will think and work better when your mind and body are working better.

- Focusing on "how" you are doing something will ultimately make the outcome of your work better.

- It takes practice to change the habits you have built up around your work environment.

- Focusing on "how" you are doing something will help you have more energy and feel better at the end of the workday.

chapter fifteen
Concepts of the Alexander Technique

We all do what we know and are familiar with, often with thoughts and preconceived ideas we don't even know we have. As you begin to understand your habits and assumptions about how you function and interface with the environment, you will discover that you can act to find your best balance and ease. As you make new choices about how you respond to a stimulus, your unique mechanism will change and support you in the best way possible, whatever activity you choose to do.

Noticing and Inhibiting
The process of paying attention to yourself and noticing how you want to respond to a stimulus (even a thought), then waiting and inhibiting your familiar response is important in changing a habit. Notice and then stop and pause. Don't do the familiar pattern simply because it might feel like the "right" thing to do.

Direction (first meaning)
In this case direction means consciously guiding and ordering yourself through a process of inserting your awareness and intention into your actions. Once you notice you are going to do an action, you can give yourself directions for how to "do" an action. Pause, redirect, and move with ease.

Direction (second meaning)
As you give yourself directions you will find a direction and flow of movement throughout your three-dimensional body. This is your body rebounding from the pull of gravity and its response will lead you to a sense of lightness, ease, and fluidity.

Ease
Allowing actions to emerge from the innate ongoing flow of energy and movement and continuing with just the amount of force needed to do the action is moving with ease. Movements and actions will then have fluidity, freedom, and balance.

fifteen: concepts of the alexander technique

End-gaining
One is end-gaining when he or she values the outcome of an action more than the process of executing the action. In other words, one emphasizes the end above the means.

Primary Control – Head, Neck, and Back Relationship
Alexander found that how the head balances on the top of the spine is primary to having better use. By releasing the neck and the downward pressure of the head on the spine, we can trigger the natural rebound from gravity throughout the entire structure. We often put pressure on ourselves by developing poor postural habits that cause us to collapse, dropping the weight of the head on the neck, down the spine and through the whole body. By releasing the downward pressure at the top of the structure the body is allowed to lengthen and widen.

chapter sixteen

Supplementary Information

F. M. Alexander (1869 - 1955)

F. M. Alexander's most significant discovery was that he caused himself to lose his voice through the way he was using his own body while orating to large audiences. Only through the close monitoring of how he was speaking was he able to change his use and eliminate his vocal problems. He further observed that his entire body responded to new ways of thinking and moving in activity and that he had come upon main principles of movement that are universal and applicable to every activity we do.

The Alexander Technique is now taught worldwide. It is particularly well established in the United States, the United Kingdom, Ireland, Germany, Switzerland, France, Canada, Australia, and Israel. It is part of the curriculum in many music, theater, and dance departments in conservatories and universities.

Alexander wrote numerous articles on his work, as well as four books:
Use of the Self
Man's Supreme Inheritance
Constructive Conscious Control of the Individual
The Universal Constant in Living

The Balance Arts Center

The Balance Arts Center, founded by Ann Rodiger, is dedicated to developing Awareness in Action – the way you think and move – through the teaching and application of the Alexander Technique.

The Balance Arts Center is based in New York city and offers a variety of ways to learn the principles of the Alexander Technique. Private instruction, group classes, and specialty workshops are all available. Balance Arts Center teachers travel to give lectures, workshops, and lessons. All ages and professions are welcome.

sixteen: supplementary information

The Balance Arts Center is also dedicated to promoting the Alexander Technique and organizes panel discussions, workshops, and conferences as well as producing products around specific topics and ideas.

People study the Alexander Technique for a variety of reasons. Some students come to refine and enhance their skills in speaking, singing, dancing, and sports while others come to work on general posture or specific ailments such as headaches, backaches, or recovery from injury.

Visit: www.balanceartscenter.com for more information.

Recommended Readings and Resources

Alexander Technique

Alexander, F. M. *Articles and Lectures*. London: Mouritz Press, 1995.

Alexander, F. M. *Constructive Conscious Control of the Individual*. London: Metheun, 1924.

Alexander, F. M. *Man's Supreme Inheritance,* 6th ed., New York: E. P. Dutton, 1941.

Alexander, F. M. *The Universal Constant in Living*. New York: E. P. Dutton, 1941.

Alexander, F. M. *Use of the Self*. New York: E. P. Dutton, 1932.

Barlow, Wilfred. *More Talk of Alexander: Aspects of the Alexander Principle*. London: Victor Gollancz, 1978.

Bloch, Michael. *F. M. The Life of Frederick Matthias Alexander*. London: Little Brown, 2004.

Caplan, Deborah, P.T. *Back Trouble: A new Approach to Prevention And Recovery*. Gainesville, FL: Triad Publishing. 1987.

Carrington, Walter. *Thinking Aloud: Talks on Teaching the Alexander Technique*. Edited by Jerry Sontag. San Francisco: Mornum Time Press, 1994.

Cranz, Galen. *The Chair*. New York: W. W. Norton, 1998.

Dart, Raymond. *Skill and Poise*. London: STAT Books, 1996.

De Alcantara, Pedro. *Indirect Procedures: A Musician's Guide to the Alexander Technique*. Oxford: Clarendon Press, 1997.

sixteen: supplementary information

Drake, Jonathan. *Body Know-how: A Practical Guide to the Use of The Alexander Technique in Everyday Life.* London: Thorsons, 1991.

Friedman, Dr. *Dr. Friedman's Vision Training Program.* New York: Bantam Books, 1983.

Gelb, Michael. *Body Learning.* New York: Delilah Books, 1981.

Grunwald, Peter. *Eyebody.* Auckland, New Zealand: Eyebody Press, 2004.

Huxley, Aldous. *Ends and Means.* New York: Harper and Brothers,1937.

Huxley, Aldous. *The Art of Seeing.* Seattle. Montana Books, 1942.

Jones, Frank Pierce. *Body Awareness in Action.* New York: Schocken Books, 1976.

Kaplan, Dr. Robert-Michael. *Seeing Beyond 20/20.* Hillsboro, OR: Beyond Words Publishing, Inc. 1987.

Langford, Elizabeth. *Mind and Muscle: An Owner's Handbook.* Apeldorn, Netherlands: Garant Uitgevers, 1998.

Maisel, Edward. *The Alexander Technique: The Essential Writings of F. Matthias Alexander.* London: Thames and Hudson, 1989.

Maisel, Edward. *The Resurrection of the Body.* New York: A Delta Book, 1974.

Park, Glen. The Art of Changing: A New Approach to the Alexander Technique. Bath: Ashgrove Press, 1989.

Sarno M.D., John E. *Healing Back Pain: The Mind-Body Connection.* New York: Warner Books, 1991.

Uppgaard, D.D.S., Robert. *Taking Control of TMJ.* Oakland, CA: New Harbinger Publications, 1999.

Vineyard, Missy. *How You Stand, How You Move, How you Live.* New York: Marlowe, 2007.

Websites

www.balanceartscenter.com
www.Balanceartscenter.blogspot.com
www.amsat.ws
www.stat.org.uk

Related Materials

Barker, Karen and Jones, Kim. *Human Movement Explained.* Oxford: Butterworth-

sixteen: supplementary information

Heinemann, 1996.

Bullock, Margaret I. *Ergonomics: The Physiotherapist in the Workplace.* Edinburgh, Churchill Livingstone, 1990.

Burke, Mike. *Ergonomics Tool Kit.* Gaithersburg, Maryland: Aspen Publications, 1998.

Calais-Germain, Blandine. *Anatomy of Movement,* Seattle: Eastland Press. 1985.

Dewey, John. *How We Think,* Amherst, NY: Prometheus Books, 1991.

Gorman, David. *The Body Moveable.* Guelph, Ontario, Canada, Ampersand Printing Co.1981.

Kapit, Wynn. *The Anatomy Coloring Book.* New York: Harper Collins, 1993.

Lane, O.D. FCVOD, Kenneth A. *Developing Ocular Motor and Visual Perception Skills.* Thorofare, NJ: Slack Inc., 2005.

Myers, Thomas W. *Anatomy Trains: Myofascial Meridians for Manual and Movement Therapists.* Edinburgh: Churchill Livingstone, 2002.

Oliver, Sherry and Bruce. *Working Without Pain: Eliminate Repetitive Strain Injuries With Alexander Technique.* Sacramento, CA, Pacific Institute for the Alexander Technique, 1997.

Pascarelli, M.D., Emil. *Complete Guide to Repetitive Strain Injury,* Hoboken, NJ: John Wiley & Sons, 2004.

Phaesant, Stephen. *Ergonomics, Work and Health.* Gaithersburg, Maryland: Aspen Publishers, Inc., 1991

Stough, Carl and Reece. *Dr. Breath.* New York: The Stough Institute, Inc., 1981.

Strozzi-Heckler, Richard. *Being Human At Work: Bringing Somatic Intelligence Into Your professional Life.* Berkeley, CA: North Atlantic Books, 2003

**For more information about the Alexander Technique contact:
Ann Rodiger at arodiger@balanceartscenter.com
or visit www.balanceartscenter.com
or call 212-439-5248.**

Also contact: www.amsat.ws

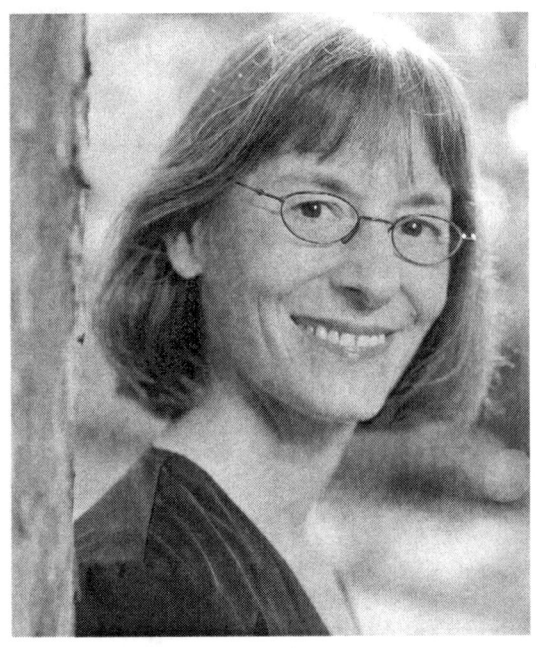

About the Author

Ann Rodiger is the founder and director of the Balance Arts Center in New York City. She is the director of the Balance Arts Center Teacher Training Course in New York City. She as been teaching the Alexander Technique for 30 years. She is also a specialist in movement education and analysis, dance, and Labanotation. She has Alexander Technique practices in New York City and Berlin, Germany. She has been on the faculty of several major universities in the United States.

CPSIA information can be obtained at www.ICGtesting.com
Printed in the USA
LVOW130953090612

285345LV00003B/1/P